Dedication

Deicated To students of obstetrics and gynecology

Acknowledgements:

I would like to acknowledge my guide Dr Mamta Rath Datta for her guidance and support. I also like to thank Dr Vishal for his help in writing my book. I like to acknowledge Dr Sonali Gulhane for providing recent information on various topics. Also I would like to thank Dr Shirin for her constant support during my residency.

Preface:

The MRCOG part 1 exam is the first step for to become obstetrician and gynecologist in UK. MRCOG is also internationally respected as the gold standard qualification for career progression in O&G. Part 1 is first step for international student to become member of Royal College of Obstetrics and Gynecology. Recently exam pattern is changed and it is consist of ONLY SBA. The exam consist of 2 paper each containing 100 SBA questions to be solved. Most of the questions in exam are clinical oriented and demand logical approach to solve them. Book will help you to know exam pattern, type of questions asked, what need to read, important point and repeatedly asked questions. I tried to cover most of important topics from basic sciences. Although exam is tough good preparation, hard work and self confidance are the key to success. This book will definitely help you to pass exam.

Dr Ankush Raut

How to read this book

Good start is half done.

"Success is not accident. It is hard work, perseverance, learning, studying, sacrifice and most of all, love of what you are doing." Pele

You must read text book on basic science in obstetrics and gynecology.

Read SBA with explanation from this book

Then read same chapter from above text book (reading SBA first will help you to know which points are important in exam point of view)

Then judge yourself by solving important questions.

Contents:

1. Biochemistry _____ 6
2. Anatomy _____ 35
3. Biophysics _____ 73
4. Clinical management _____ 79
5. Embryology _____ 85
6. Endocrinology _____ 104
7. Cell _____ 118
8. Microbiology _____ 122
9. Pathology _____ 152
10. Pharmacology _____ 175
11. Physiology _____ 194

1.Biochemistry

1. Cell membrane primarily composed of:
   a) Phosphatidylcholine
   b) Phosphatidylethanolamine
   c) Phosphatidylinisitol
   d) Phosphatidylserine
   e) All of above
   Answer: e

The plasma membrane comprised primarily of Phospholipid bilayers. There are four major Types of phospholipid (phosphatidyl-choline, ethanolamine, -inositol, and -serine), each formed by esterification of two fatty acyl chains (typically one saturated and one polyunsaturated fatty acid) to a glycerol backbone with the polar/ charged head group attached to the third carbon of that glycerol skeleton. Due to the hydrophobic nature of the fatty acyl tails, Which form the core of the phospholipid bilayer, polar .Compounds (e.g. Glucose) and charged ions (e.g. $Na +$, $k +$, $cl -$, and $HCO 3 -$) are unable to pass across the membrane bilayer without a protein-based transport mechanism. Hence, phospholipids effectively insulate cells (and their constituent organelles), allowing them to selectively take up or exclude specific hydrophilic molecules and ions, creating specific microenvironments within the cell. The Typical cell membrane also contains two additional components: cholesterol and membrane proteins. Cholesterol increases membrane fluidity to the extent that the ultimate hydrophilic molecule, water, can pass through small spaces between neighboring phospholipid molecules without destabilizing the membrane.

By virtue of its molecular structure, at low to medium Concentrations, cholesterol decreases the Van Der Waal's forces and hydrogen bonding between adjacent lipid molecules, so increasing membrane fluidity. At high concentrations cholesterol paradoxically decreases membrane fluidity, as the cholesterol molecules become organized into a stable, semicrystalline structure. Proteins either reside within the cell membrane ('integral' membrane proteins) or associate with the hydrophilic head groups of the phospholipid molecules ('peripheral' membrane Proteins). Membrane proteins typically serve as transport proteins, enzymes, or receptors.

Cytoplasmic proteins that are not associated with the cell membrane can make similar structural and functional contributions in the cytoplasm of the cell.

1. Fuel of cell is:
   a) CPK
   b) ATP
   c) CDP
   d) MLK
   e) All of above
      Answer: b

2. Michaelis-menten(Km) constant is:
   a) Amount of substrate at v max
   b) Substrate concentration at ½ vmax
   c) Velocity of reaction
   d) Always constant for every reaction
   e) All of above
      Answer: b

Assuming first order enzyme kinetics, the Michaelis-Menten constant (Km) is the substrate concentration at which the reaction reaches a velocity equal to half of the maximal rate (V max /2).

3. Under aerobic condition all respiratory substance end in :
   a) Glycolysis
   b) Glyconeogenisis
   c) Citric acid cycle
   d) Pentose pathway
   e) Fatty acid oxidation

Answer: c

Under aerobic conditions, all respiratory substrates ultimately end up in the Krebs cycle (also known as the citric acid or Tricarboxylic acid cycle).

4. Oxidative phosphorylation occurs in:
   a) Outer mitochondrial membrane.
   b) Inner mitochondrial membrane
   c) Endoplasmic reticulum
   d) Golgi apparatus
   e) Nucleus

Answer: b

The oxidative phosphorylation pathway comprises four sequential protein complexes, acting in concert with ATP synthase embedded in the inner mitochondrial membrane.

5. Process that established concentration gradient across inner mitochondrial membrane is called
   a) Chemiosmosis
   b) Osmosis
   c) Citric acid cycle
   d) HMP pathway
   e) Fatty acid oxidation

Answer: a

Complexes I, III, and IV each export protons from the mitochondrial matrix into the aqueous space between the inner and the outer mitochondrial membranes in a process termed chemiosmosis. This establishes a concentration/Ph gradient across the inner mitochondrial membrane and it is the flux of protons down this gradient back into the matrix via ATP synthase that drives the phosphorylation of ADP to ATP.

6. Complex I passes electron to:
   a) Ubiquinol
   b) FAD
   c) Cytochrome c reductase
   d) Cytochrome
   e) Cytochrome c oxidase

Answer: a

Complex I (NADH dehydrogenase or NADH-coenzyme Q oxidoreductase) binds NADH and oxidizes this back to NAD + (and a proton). The abstracted pair of electrons passes via a Flavin mononucleotide (FMN) prosthetic group to Iron-Sulphur (Fe-S) centres in complex I and ultimately on to ubiquinone (coenzyme q), which is reduced to ubiquinol.

As the electrons pass through complex I, protons bind to the matrix face of the complex and are transferred across to be liberated into the intermembrane space.

• complex II, which comprises four protein subunits and incorporates succinate dehydrogenase (succinate coenzyme Q oxidoreductase), does not lie downstreamof complex I, but instead represents an independent point of entry into the oxidative phosphorylation pathway . This complex contains FAD bound within the Inner mitochondrial membrane, and as the dehydrogenase component oxidizes succinate to fumarate, the hydrogen ions pass to this nucleotide co-factor, reducing the FAD to FADH2 . Within complex II, the electrons again pass via Fe-S centres to coenzyme Q/ubiquinone, but because complex II does not span the inner mitochondrial membrane, any protons bound by this complex have to be returned to the mitochondrial matrix (rather than being exported into the aqueous inter-membrane space).

• From complexes I and II, the electrons pass via ubiquinol to complex III (cytochrome c reductase): a dimeric assembly wherein each monomer contains 11 protein subunits associated with a single cytochrome c molecule and two b cytochromes. Each of the cytochromes contains at least one haem group in which the iron can either accept or donate electrons (transiting between the Fe2 + and Fe 3 + states, respectively). As a consequence, complex III is able to receive electrons from complexes I and II (recycling the ubiquinol back to ubiquinone) and to pass those electrons on to cytochrome c. As the electrons pass through complex III, protons are bound on the Matrix side of the complex and are exported into the Intermembrane space (as for complex I).

The final complex of the oxidative phosphorylationPathway, complex IV (cytochrome c oxidase), comprises 13 protein subunits, two haem groups, and ionic copper (Cu + /Cu 2 +), magnesium, and zinc. By virtue of its transition metal ions, complex IV can accept the electrons from the haem groups of cytochrome c (which then relax from their Fe2 + to the Fe3 + state). The electrons pass through complex IV to oxygen in the mitochondrial matrix, which splits into oxide ions and recombines with protons to form water molecules. As complex IV transports electrons and forms water, it also provides the third opportunity for protons to be exported from the mitochondrial matrix into the intermembrane space.

7. Oligomycin inhibits:
   a) Complex i
   b) Complex ii
   c) Cytochrome c reductase
   d) F_0
   e) Cytochrome c oxidase

Answer: d

like complexes I,III, and IV (but not complex ii), ATP synthase also spans the inner mitochondrial membrane. F_0 region of ATP synthase spans the membrane while the globular F1 domain, which contains the synthase enzyme, protrudes into the mitochondrial matrix. As the protons exported into the intermembrane space of the mitochondrion by complexes I, III, and IV re-enter the matrix along the proton channel in the f domain, they provide energy to the f 1 domain required to power the synthesis of the high-energy, terminal phosphate bond in ATP. Some antibiotics, such as oligomycin, inhibit the f 0 domain of ATP synthase, which contributes to the lethargic side effects of such drugs.

8. $FADH_2$ produce_____ no of ATP molecule:
   a) 3
   b) 2
   c) 4
   d) 5
   e) 1

Answer: b

Since NADH enters the oxidative phosphorylationPathway at complex I, there are three opportunities to Export protons from the mitochondrial matrix (via complexes I, III, and IV) such that each molecule of NADH produced in the metabolism of a respiratory substrate generates up to three molecules of ATP. However, when succinate is oxidized by succinate dehydrogenase in complex II, protons can only be exported via complexes III and IV. Consequently, the oxidation of FADH 2 back to FAD can only power the synthesis of two molecules of ATP.

TCA cycle: - **Oxaloacitic acid** combines with **acetyl –CoA** and converted into **citrate** in presence of enzyme **citrate synthase**.

- Then aconitase act on citrate and dehydrolyse citrate results in formation of **isocitrate** and one molecule of water.

- isocitrate combines with NAD in presence of isocitrate dehydrogenase results in formation of NADH2, **alpha ketoglutarate** and water molecule.

- alpha keto-glutarate converted into **succinyl Co-A** and NADH2 form in presence of alpha keto glutarate dehydrogenase.

- then succinyl CoA undergo substrate level phosphorylation and form 1 molecule of **GTP** from GDP with succinate as terminal molecule in presence of succinyl Co A synthtase

- succinate then act ny succinate dehydrogenase and release **FADH2** and **Fumarate.**

- fumarate is act by fumarase and L-Malate is form which further converted into Oxaloacitic acid(OAA) in presence of malate dehydrogenase with release of NADH2.

- With formation of OAA cycle further repeated.

Electron transport chain:
There two gate ways for H2 go into cycle:
Through succinate Q-reductase : FADH2 enters like this and 2 ATP molecule is form.
FADH2 give electron to succinate Q reductase which pass electron to Ubiquinone which then pass to cytochrome

reductase – cytochrome C – cytochrome oxidase finally O2 and water is formed.

Through NADH2 Pathway three molecules of ATP are formed. Electron enters from NADH-Q reductase and pass to Ubiquinone . remaining pathway is same as above after ubiquinone.

9. Each turn of kreb's cycle produce_____ATP:
   a) 12
   b) 14
   c) 10
   d) 6
   e) 1

Answer: a

10. FADH$_2$ produce by:
    a) Isocitrate dehydrogenase
    b) Alpha keto glutarate dehydrogenase
    c) Succinate dehydrogenase
    d) Malate dehydrogenase
    e) Succinyl CO-A synthtase

Answer: c

11. Substrate level phosphorylation is at lelvel:
    a) Isocitrate dehydrogenase
    b) Alpha keto glutarate dehydrogenase
    c) Succinate dehydrogenase
    d) Malate dehydrogenase
    e) Succinyl CoA synthtase

Answer: e

The Krebs cycle (or tricarboxylic acid/TCA cycle) operates in the mitochondrial matrix only **under aerobic conditions.**

In the initial rate-limiting formation of citrate, the 2carbonAcetate is attached to Coenzyme A via a sulphurous Thioester linkage as Acetyl-CoA. Cleavage of the high-energy thioester bond in Acetyl-CoA provides the energy for the formation of the new carbon-carbon bond when the acetate is combined with the oxaloacetate by the enzyme citrate synthase to form citrate. After this aconitase converts citrate to isocitrate via the metabolic intermediate, aconitate. Isocitrate oxidized by Isocitrate dehydrogenase to form the five carbon (5c) metabolite, alpha-ketoglutarate ,this reaction liberate CO2 and $NADH_2$,which will ultimately contribute to the ATP yield of this metabolic cycle . The very next reaction, catalized by alpha-ketoglutarate dehydrogenase which convert alpha-ketoglutarate to succinyl CoA along with production of CO_2 and $NADH_2$ Succinyl CoA synthtase convert succinyl CoA to Succinate along with production of GTP. This molecule is the only one to be generated in the Krebs cycle by substrate-level phosphorylation independently of the mitochondrial oxidative phosphorylation pathway.

Succinate is oxidized to Fumarate by succinate dehydrogenase , reducing FAD to FADH 2 . **While seven of the eight enzymes of the krebs cycle exist within the matrix of the mitochondrion, succinate dehydrogenase is unusual in being embedded in the inner mitochondrial**. Membrane where it constitutes an integral part of Complex II of the oxidative phosphorylation pathway.

Fumarate is then hydrated by fumarase to form malate then malate dehydrogenase oxidizes the malate to oxaloacetate, reducing NAD + to $NADH_2$ in the process. Each turn of the Krebs cycle can generate up to 12 molecules of ATP.

12. In aerobic condition glucose produce_____ATP:
    a) 2
    b) 8
    c) 38
    d) 30
    e) 109

Answer: c

13. In anaerobic condition glucose produce_____ATP:
    a) 2
    b) 8
    c) 38
    d) 30

e) 109

Answer: b

14. In anaerobic condition glucose net gain of ATP is:

a) 8
b) 38
c) 30
d) 109
e) 2

Answer: e

15. Insulin dependant glucose uptake(GLUT 4) occur in:

a) Fetal tessue
b) Brain
c) RBC
d) Skeletal muscle
e) All of above

Answer: d

Glycolysis relies on the cellular uptake of glucose from extracellular fluid/plasma. Glucose is hydrophilic and so cannot diffuse freely across cell membranes. So require protein transporter. Following membrane uptake, glucose oxidation through the glycolytic pathway occurs in the cytosol.

In fetal tissues, adult erythrocytes, and the brain, glucose uptake is mediated via the low affinity, high capacity GLUT 1 protein. In skeletal muscle and adipose tissue, glucose uptake occurs via the insulin-sensitive GLUT4 transporter.

Although glycolysis can occur in the absence of oxygen (i.e. Under anaerobic conditions, and in cells that lack mitochondria such as red blood cells), this reaction series generates a relatively modest yield of reduced nucleotide co-factors, and hence of ATP. (of the maximum net gain of 38 molecules of ATP generated through the aerobic oxidation of each molecule of glucose, only eight molecules are generated through glycolysis; this decreases to a net gain of **only two molecules of ATP per molecule of Glucose respired under anaerobic conditions.**

16. ATP dependent reaction in glycolysis catalyze by:
    a) Hexokinase
    b) 6-phosphofructokinase
    c) Aldolase
    d) Glyceraldehyde phosphate dehydrogenase
    e) Both a and b

Answer: e

17. In glycolsis substrate level phosphorylation occur at:
    a) Hexokinase
    b) 6-phosphofructokinase
    c) Pyruvate kinase
    d) Phosphoglycerate kinase
    e) C and d

Answer: e

18. In glycolsis $NADH_2$ produce at level of:
    a) Hexokinase
    b) 6-phosphofructokinase
    c) Pyruvate kinase
    d) Glyceraldehyde phosphate dehydrogenase
    e) Enolase

Answer: d

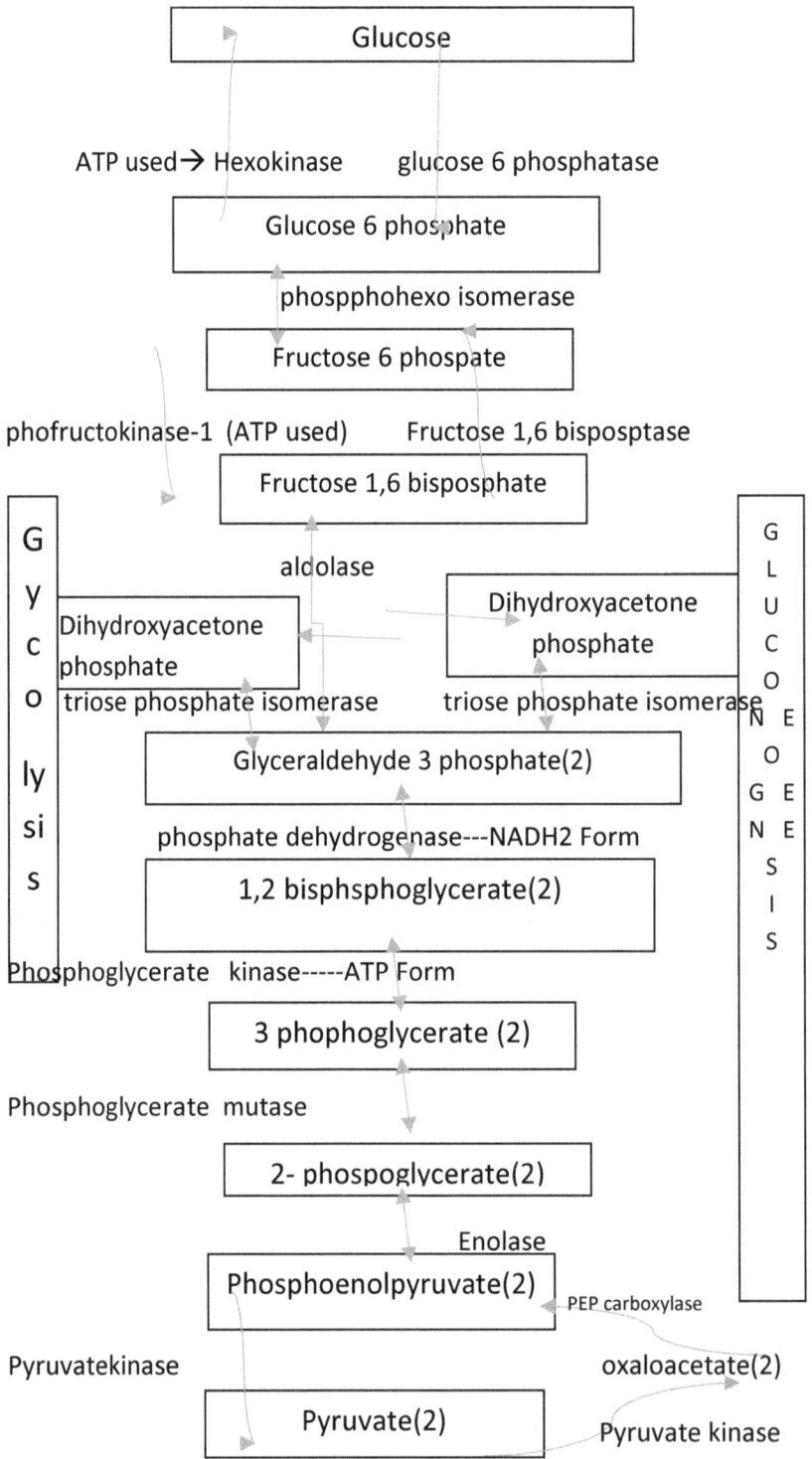

19. In order to take part in Kreb's cycle pyruvate must be converted into:
    a) Acetyl CoA
    b) Oxaloacetate
    c) Citrate
    d) Alpha ketoglutarate
    e) Malate

Answer: a

Alternative fates of pyruvate

pyruvate   *lactate dehydrogenase*   lactate +NAD$^+$
+
NADH

pyruvate   *pyruvate dehydrogenase*   *acetyl coa*
+   +NADH +CO$_2$
NAD$^+$ + CoA-SH

pyruvate   *pyruvate carboxylase*   oxaloacetate
+
CO$_2$

20. End product of oxidation of fatty acid containing odd number of carbon is:
    a) Acetyl CoA
    b) Propionyl CoA
    c) Citrate
    d) Alpha ketoglutarate
    e) Malate

Answer: b

Beta-oxidation cycle

The beta-oxidation cycle, which occurs in the mitochondrial matrix, is the literative cleavage of 2carbon fragments from a fatty acid chain to generate Acetyl-CoA molecules that enter the krebs cycle.in the case of fatty acids containing even numbers of carbon atoms, the betaoxidation cycle converts the fatty acid exclusively into 2C acetyl groups (seven, eight, or nine Acetyl-CoA molecules per molecule of myristic, palmitic, or stearic acid, respectively). For odd numbered fatty acids, 2c subunits are cleaved until the final 3c fragment remains as a propionyl-CoA molecule, i.e. The rare 17c fatty acid margaric acid would undergo the beta-oxidation cycle to yield seven (rather than eight) acetyl- CoA molecules and a single propionyl-CoA molecule. The propionyl grouping has the same problem entering the Krebs cycle as pyruvate: the propionyl group has three carbons, and three is not a number favoured by the Krebs cycle. Therefore, any propionyl-coa formed by beta-oxidation of odd-chain fatty acids must be carboxylated to enter the krebs cycle as the 4c component of succinyl-CoA (which decreases the ATP yield of propionyl-CoA to only six ATP per turn of the krebs cycle, as opposed to 12 ATP per turn for each Acetyl-CoA molecule).

21. In beta-oxidation of fatty acid acyl CoA is transported from cytosol to mitochondria by:
    a) CPT i
    b) CPTi
    c) Pyruvate dehydrogenase
    d) Thiolase
    e) Hydrolase

Answer: a

22. In beta-oxidation of fatty acid acyl CoA number of $NADH_2$ and $FADH_2$ produce are
    a) 1,2
    b) 1,1
    c) 0,2
    d) 2,0
    e) 0,0

Answer: b

The beta-oxidation cycle is preceded by esterification of a 'free' or non-esterified fatty acid (NEFA) chain onto the sulphydryl/thiol group of coenzyme a to form a Fatty Acyl-CoA molecule. (this is important since the Thioester bond provides the energy to power this metabolic cycle.)

There then follows a series of four reactions, and in each round the length of the fatty Acyl-CoA molecule is decreased by two carbons.First two reactions are oxidation reaction where $NADH_2$ and $FADH_2$ is produce. This has two consequences. Firstly, it means that beta-oxidation of fatty acids leads to the generation of ATP prior to the entry of the Acetyl-CoA fragments into the Krebs cycle. Secondly, this requirement for FAD and NAD + to be recycled (via the oxidative phosphorylation pathway) **explains why fat metabolism can only occur during aerobic conditions.**

Fatty Acyl-CoA is formed in the cytosol of the cell, whereas the beta-oxidation cycle occurs within the mitochondrial matrix. In order to pass across the aqueous space between the mitochondrial membranes, cytosolic Acyl-CoA combine with carnitine at the outer mitochondrial membrane, catalysed by the carnitine palmitoyl transferase (CPT) I enzyme, and then released by the action of CPT II in the inner mitochondrial membrane.

Beta oxiadation of fatty acid

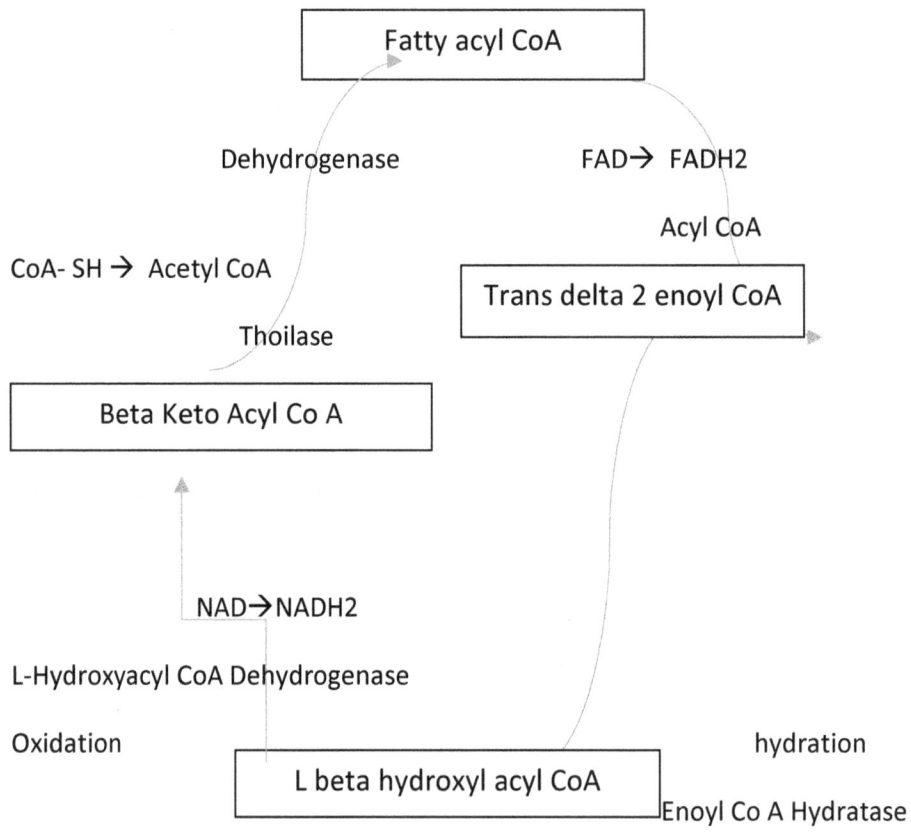

23. Ketone bodies are produce in:
    a) Liver
    b) Brain
    c) Kidney
    d) Stomach
    e) Pancrease

Answer: a
24. Ketone bodies are :
    a) 3-hydroxybuterate
    b) Acetoacetate
    c) Both a and b

d) Oxaloacitate

e) Pyruvate

Answer: c

For Acetyl CoA liver beta-oxidation . In specific metabolic conditions (e.g. Starvation), hepatic beta-oxidation generates more Acetyl-CoA than can be incorporated into the Krebs cycle. Within the hepatic mitochondria, the excess Acetyl-CoA molecules can be combined (by thiolase) to generate Acetoacetyl-CoA molecules, which can be coupled with Acetyl-CoA to synthesize 3-hydroxy-3-methylglutaryl-CoA. Cleavage of this product by HMGA lyase liberates Acetyl-CoA and free acetoacetate, where the latter can be reduced to 3-hydroxybutyrate by the reversible 3-hydroxybutyrate dehydrogenase enzyme.Acetoacetate and 3-hydroxybutyrate, collectively termed 'ketone bodies', are exported into the circulation and taken up by extra-hepatic tissues, most importantly the brain and skeletal muscle, where they serve as respiratory substrates. Hydroxybutyrate can be oxidized back to acetoacetate which is converted to Acetyl-CoA (via an acetoacetyl-coa intermediate) to fuel the Krebs cycle

25. Which of following is water soluble vitamin:

a) A

b) D

c) E

d) K

e) B1

Answer: e

26. Night blindness is caused deficiency of:

a) A

b) D

c) E

d) K

e) B1

Answer: a

27. Rickets is caused deficiency of:

a) A

b) Pre-pubertal deficiency of vitamin d

c) Post-pubertal deficiency of vitamin d

d) K

e) B1

Answer: b

28. Which of following vitamin act as antioxidant and its deficiency cause mild hemolytic anemia in newborn

a) A

b) D

c) E

d) K

e) B1

Answer: c

29. Deficiency of following deficiency cause bleeding diathesis

a) A

b) D

c) E

d) K

e) B1

Answer: d

30. Deficiency of following vitamin cause beriberi:

a) A

b) D

c) E

d) K

e) B1

Answer: d

31. Deficiency of following vitamin deficiency cause Arbinoflevinosis

a) A

b) D

c) Riboflavin

d) K

e) B1

Answer: c

32. Deficiency of following vitamin deficiency cause pellagra

a) A

b) D

c) B2

d) B3

e) B1

Answer: d

33. Deficiency of following vitamin deficiency cause paraesthesia:

a) B2

b) B3

c) Pantothenic acid

d) K

e) B1

Answer: c

34. Overdose of following vitamin deficiency cause impairment of neurological function:

a) B2

b) B3

c) Pantothenic acid

d) Pyridoxin

e) B1

Answer: d

35. Deficiency of following vitamin deficiency cause dermatitis enteritis :

a) B2

b) B3

c) Pantothenic acid

d) Biotin

e) B1

Answer: d

36. Deficiency of following vitamin deficiency cause scurvy:

a) A

b) C

c) Pantothenic acid

d) K

e) B1

Answer: b

37. Deficiency of following vitamin deficiency cause megaloblastic anemia:

a) B9

b) B12

c) Pantothenic acid

d) Both a and b

e) B1

Answer: d

38. Diarrhea caused by overdose of:

a) B2

b) B3

c) C

d) K

e) B1

Answer: c

39. In starvation brain mostly use:

a) Glucose

b) Fructose

c) Ketone bodies

d) Glycogen

e) Amino acid

Answer: c

1. Brain, rely on glucose (or, in starvation, on ketone bodies) as their energy source. **2.** Although it is possible to metabolize excess glucose into fatty acids (and hence to triglyceride), it is never possible to reverse this reaction; fatty acids cannot be used to derive glucose. **3.** Once glycogen stores have been depleted, the supply of plasma glucose for brain activity can be maintained by using the carbon skeletons of amino acids (never fatty acids).

40. Glycogen is mainly stored in:
   a) Liver
   b) Skeletal muscle
   c) Brain
   d) Both a and b
   e) Uterus

Answer: d

Glycogen ('animal starch') is a polysaccharide formed by the sequential polymerization of glucose molecules primarily through alpha 1,4-glycosidic bonds. Approximately 8 % of the glucose molecules are added via alpha-1,6-glycosidic bonds, which creates branch points in the glycogen molecule . The synthesis of glycogen is catalyzed by glycogen synthase, an anabolic enzyme that is stimulated after a meal by insulin (and inhibited in the fasting state byHormones such as glucagon and adrenaline).

• glycogen is stored primarily in the liver and skeletal muscle (where insulin stimulates glucose uptake via the GLUT4 glucose transporter).

41. Glycogenolysis catalyzed by:
   a) Glycogen phosphorylase
   b) Glycogen synthase
   c) Glycogen reductase
   d) Glucose 6 phosphotase
   e) Glucose 1 phosphotase

Answer: a

42. In starvation glucose from glycogen release by:
   a) Liver

b) Brain

c) Pancreas

d) Gall blader

e) Kidney

Answer: a

43. In glycogenolysis glycogen converted into:

a) Glucose 1phosphate

b) Glucose 6 phosphate

c) Glucose 1,6 phosphate

d) Glucose

e) Fructose

Answer: b>a

The catabolism of glycogen, termed glycogenolysis(not to be confused with 'glycolysis'), is catalysed by the enzyme glycogen phosphorylase, which acts sequentially to liberate glucose-1-phosphate molecules from the glycogen, shortening the glycogen polymer by 1 glucose subunit. The glucose-1-phosphate is then isomerized to glucose-6-phosphate by phosphoglucomutase.

Since the charged glucose-6-phosphate molecule cannot pass across the plasma membrane of the cells, in most tissues (including the vagina, uterus, and skeletal muscle) glucose-6-phosphate generated by glycogenolysis has to be metabolized (by glycolysis) within the very same cell that held the glycogen store.

Only hepatocytes express the glucose-6-phosphatase enzyme required to remove the phosphate ion, and so only the liver can export glucose into the bloodstream to support glycolysis (and the Krebs cycle) at distant sites.

44. In fasting state cortisol must upregulates:

a) Phosphoenolpyruvate carboxykinase

b) Fructose 1,6 biphosphatase

c) Glucose 6 phosphotase

d) Pyruvate carboxylase

e) All of above

Answer: e

45. In prolonged fasting state there is:

a) Utilization of glucose

b) Utilization of fat

c) Mobilization of glycogen

d) Mobilization of amino acid

e) None of above

Answer: d

In the fasted state, cortisol must up-regulate
The expression of three gluconeogenic enzymes:
1. Phosphoenolpyruvate carboxykinase (PEPCK) —
Required to metabolize oxaloacetate to phosphoenolpyruvate **2.**
Fructose-1,6-bisphosphatase — required to catalyse the
dephosphorylation of fructose-1,6-bisphosphate to fructose-6-
phosphate
3. Glucose-6-phosphatase — required to hydrolyse glucose- 6-
phosphate to free glucose (for export fromThe liver).
• in addition, cortisol increases the expression of pyruvate
carboxylase (to increase the metabolism of pyruvate to
oxaloacetate) and the enzymes of the urea cycle (required to
process the ammonium liberated when amino acids are
converted into keto acids for the Krebs cycle).

46. In anaerobic fasting state:

a) Only glycolytic pathway is effective

b) Accumulation of lactate

c) Decrease in intracellular ph

d) Lactate oxidized by Cori`s cycle to pyruvate

e) All of above

Answer: e

Under anaerobic conditions, effective metabolic pathway is
glycolytic pathway. Which produce lactic acid along with small
amount of ATP. Lactic acid decrease Ph.

Important questions:

1. Essential amino acid among following is :
   a) Alanine
   b) Tyrosine
   c) Serine
   d) Tryptophan
   e) Proline
   Answer: d

1. Basic   amino acid among following is :
   a) Aspartic acid
   b) Glutamic acid
   c) Asparagine
   d) Arginine
   e) Glutamine
   Answer: d

2. Aliphatic chain amino acid among following are :
   a) Alanine
   b) Glycin
   c) Valin
   d) Leucine
   e) All of above
   Answer: e

3. Process of transcription produce:
   a) rRNA
   b) tRNA
   c) mRNA
   d) DNA
   e) Protein
   Answer: c

4. Techniques use for protein separation are:
   a) Gel permeation chromatography
   b) Gel electrophorasis
   c) Ion exchange chromatography
   d) Affinity chromatography

e) All of above

Answer: e

5. Single molecule of glucose will produce
   a) 30 ATP
   b) 38 ATP
   c) 40 ATP
   d) 48 ATP
   e) 7300 cal

   Answer: b

6. False statement regarding glycolysis is:
   a) Net gain of reaction is 2 ATP and 2 NADH molecule
   b) In aerobic condition total 8 ATP produce
   c) 2 ATP are consumed in early stage of cycle
   d) Cannot work in anaerobic condition
   e) In anaerobic condition pyruvate is converted into lactic acid

   Answer: d

7. Which of the following enzyme in TCA produce $FADH_2$
   a) Iso-citrate dehydrogenase
   b) Alpha- ketoglutarate dehdrogenase
   c) Malate dehydrogenase
   d) Succinate thiokinase
   e) Succinate dehydrogenase

   Answer: e

8. For glucose estimation bulb containing sodium fluoride is use because it inhibits:
   a) Enolase
   b) Pyruvate kinase
   c) Glyceraldehyde dehydrogenase
   d) Phosphoglycerate kinase
   e) Aldolase

   Answer: a

9. Fluoroacetate inhibit:
   a) Aconitase

b) Isocitrate dehydrogenase

c) Fumarase

d) Succinate dehydrogenase

e) Alpha glutarate dehydrogenase

Answer: a

10. Complex ii of respiratory chain is inhibited by:

a) Rotenone

b) Antimycin a

c) Cyanide

d) Malonate

e) 2,4 dinitrophenol

Answer: d

11. Fatty acid essential for health are:

a) Linoleic acid

b) Linolenic acid

c) Arachidonic acid

d) All of above

e) Only a and b

Answer d

12. In the first two days of starvation energy is mostly derived from:

a) Fatty acid oxidation

b) Break down of tissue protein

c) Glycogenolysis

d) Gluconeogenesis

e) Both c and d

Answer: e

13. Ketone bodies are detected by:

a) Rothera`s test

b) Benedict`s test

c) Hay sulphur test

d) Fouchet`s test

e) Salvinoff`s test

Answer: a

14. Half life of RBC is:

a) 100 days
b) 120 days
c) 140 days
d) 120 hours
e) 120 weeks
Answer: b

15. In erythropioetic porphyria there is deficiency of:
a) Ferrochelatase
b) Uroporphyrinogen i synthtase
c) Proto porphyrinogen oxidase
d) Coproprophyrinogen oxidase
e) Uroporphyrinogen iii synthtase
Answer: a

16. Amino acid which is intermediate for metabolism of all amino acid is:
a) Citrullin
b) Glutamic acid
c) Arginosuccinate
d) Arginine
e) Ornithine
Answer: b

17. Urea cycle mostly takes place in:
a) Kidney
b) Intestine
c) Pancreas
d) Liver
e) Brain
Answer: d

18. Brain cannot produce urea due to deficiency of:
a) Carbamoyl PO4 synthtase
b) Ornithine carbamoyl transferase
c) Arginosuccinic acid synthtase
d) Arginosuccinase
e) Arginase
Answer: b

19. Proteins are denatured by
    a) Heating
    b) Change in ph
    c) Organic solvant
    d) Radiation
    e) All of above
       Answer: e

20. Wrong statement among following is:
    a) Michaelis constant is the concentration of substance at which velocity of reaction is maximal .
    b) In competitive inhibition Km increased while Vmax remain is unaltered
    c) In non competitive inhibition Km remain same but Vmax is reduced
    d) In non competitive inhibition inhibitor bind at the same place at which substrate bind
    e) Lineweaver-burk plot is used for Vmax and Km ploting
       Answer: d

21. Water soluble vitamin is:
    a) A
    b) D
    c) B
    d) E
    e) K
       Answer: c

22. False statement among following;
    a) Chief cell secrete pepsinogen which converted into pepsin by HCl secreted by parietal cell(oxyntic cell)
    b) Pepsin cause peptide bond hydrolysis next to tryptophan , phenylalanine, tyrosine (aromatic amino acid)

c) Trypsinogen is activated by enterokinase which in turn activate procarboxypeptidase and chymotrypsinogen

d) Trypsin cleave peptide bond next to acidic amino acid

e) Microvilli of intestine contain peptidase which convert di and tri peptidase into single amino acid

Answer:d

23. Regarding carbohydrate metabolism
a) Most common carbohydrate in diet is starch
b) Starch break down into maltose and isomaltose by salivary and pancreatic amylase
c) Mucosal villi contain maltase , isomaltase , lactase, sucrase which break down maltose isomaltose lactate and sucrose into monosaccharide
d) Glucose and galactose absorb by active process and fructose absorb by passive process
e) All of above true
Answer: e

24. Emulsification of fat is done by:
a) Urea
b) Bile salt
c) Amylase
d) Peptidase
e) Cholecystokinin
Answer: b

25. False statement among following is:
a) Arachodonic acid is produce by action of phospholipase a 2 phospholipase c diacylglycerol lipases
b) Cox i is constitutively expressed
c) Cox ii is inducible and responsible for infection and preterm labour

d) PGF-2-aplha used for treatment of preterm labour

e) Low dose aspirin mainly inhibit thromboxane synthesis in platelet permanently with little effect on vascular endothelial prostacyclin synthesis

Answer: d

26. Indomethacin mainly inhibits following enzyme in treatment of menorrhagia and preterm labour:

a) COX i

b) COX ii

c) Thromboxane synthtase

d) Lipo-oxgnase

e) Diacyl glycerol lipase

Answer: b

27. Following statement is false about nitric oxide

a) E-NOS is calcium calmodulin dependent and relaxes smooth muscle, prevent aggregation of platelets

b) NOS I is calcium calmodulin independent and produce by macrophages and neutrophil

c) B neutrophil is produce by brain and calcium calmodulin complex dependent

d) NO is responsible for penile errection

e) None of above

Answer: e

2.Anatomy:

1. Function of anterior abdominal wall muscle are:
   a) Flex trunk
   b) Act as accessory muscle for respiration
   c) Help in defecation, micturition, parturation
   d) Protect abdominal organ from trauma
   e) All of above
      Answer: e

2. Posterior rectus sheath is absent in:
   a) Below arcuate line
   b) Over 5 to 7 coastal cartilage
   c) Between umbilicus to pubic crest
   d) Above arcuate line
   e) Both a and b
      Answer: e

Rectus abdominis
• This arises from the pubic crest and inserts into the fifth to seventh costal cartilages. Its outlines can easily be defined in subjects of normal build by the midline linea alba and the linea semilunaris along its curved lateral border when the abdominal muscles are tensed.
• It is contained within the fibrous rectus sheath, formed in the main by a split in the aponeurosis of the internal oblique muscle.
• Posteriorly this is reinforced by the aponeurosis of the transversus abdominis and anteriorly by the external oblique.
• Below a level halfway between the umbilicus and the pubic crest, demarcated by the rather ill-defined arcuate line of douglas, the aponeuroses all pass in front of the rectus. This gap enables the inferior epigastric vessels, which arise from the external illiacs, to pass upwards into the posterior sheath.
• Above the costal margin the posterior sheath is also absent; the uppermost part of the rectus abdominis lies directly against, and attached to, the fifth to seventh costal cartilages. Here the anterior sheath is made up entirely of the aponeurosis of the external oblique.

3. Inguinal ligament which extend from superior iliac spine to pubic tubercle represents:
   a) Rolled out lower border of external oblique aponeurosis
   b) Rolled out lower border of internal oblique aponeurosis
   c) Rolled out lower border of transverse abdominus
   d) Both a and b
   e) All of above

   Answer: a

The lateral muscles
Above the level of the iliac crest, the fibers of the *external oblique* muscle pass downwards and medially, those of the *internal oblique* pass upwards and forwards, and those of the *transverses abdominis* run transversely. Below this line, these muscles become aponeurotic and their fibers pass downwards and medially in the formation of the inguinal Canal.

• The *inguinal ligament* , passing from the anterior superior iliac spine to the pubic tubercle, represents the rolled lower border of the external oblique aponeurosis.

4. In Lerich syndrome anastomosis between superior and inferior epigastric artery connects:
   a) Subclavian and internal iliac artery
   b) Subclavian and external iliac artery
   c) Femoral and internal iliac artery
   d) Femoral and external iliac artery
   e) None of above

   Answer: b

5. Anterior abdominal wall is innervated by:
   a) Posterior primary rami of t7 to 11
   b) Anterior primary rami of t7 to 11
   c) Anterior primary rami of t9 to 11
   d) Posterior primary rami of t9 to 11
   e) None of above

   Answer: b

6. Spinal anesthesia is given for elective LSCS, surgeon check for level of anesthesia by at level of umbilicus. Umbilicus correspond to
   a) T7
   b) T10
   c) L1
   d) T4
   e) L4

   Answer: b

7. Suprapubic skin is supplied by:
   a) Iliohypogastric nerve
   b) Genitofemoral nerve
   c) Ilioinguinal
   d) Femoral
   e) Obturator

   Answer: a

Blood supply

The anterior abdominal wall : lower intercostals and subcostal vessels. In addition, the inferior epigastric vessels, which anastomose with the smaller superior epigastric artery and vein, the terminal branches of the internal thoracic vessels. This arterial anastomosis is an important communication between the subclavian artery above and the external iliac artery below, for example in occlusion of the lower aorta (Leriche syndrome) and in coarctation of the aorta. Of more immediate concern is that these vessels may be lacerated at insertion of the lateral trocar at laparoscopy.

Nerve supply

The anterior abdominal wall is innervated by the anterior primary rami of T7 to L1. The cutaneous segmental supply is easily mapped out on the patient — T7 supplies the xiphoid region, **T10 the level of the umbilicus, and L1 the groin.** L1 divides on the posterior abdominal wall to form the iliohypogastric and ilioinguinal nerves. The former runs deep to the external oblique just above the inguinal canal to supply the suprapubic skin, while the latter traverses the inguinal canal in front of the round ligament. It emerges either through the external inguinal ring or through the adjacent aponeurosis to supply the skin of the anterior part of the labium majus together with the skin of the adjacent upper thigh.

8. False statement about Pfannensteil's incision is
   a) Given 2 cm above pubic symphysis
   b) Peritoneum is separated superiorly
   c) Rectus sheath is separated from rectus muscle upto umbilicus above
   d) Rectus sheath separated from rectus muscle upto pubic symphysis below
   e) Bladder must be empty

Answer: a

• *The Pfannensteil incision:* a curving interspinous skin crease incision is made about 5 cm above the pubis just inferior to the margin of the pubic hair line. The anterior rectus sheath is divided to its full extent at this level on each side and dissected off the adherent underlying rectus muscle almost to the umbilicus above and to the pubis below. The recti are then retracted laterally, exposing the peritoneum covered by a variable amount of extraperitoneal fascia. As with the lower midline incision, the peritoneum is opened at the superior end of the incision to ensure that the bladder (which should first invariably be emptied by a catheter) is not wounded.

9. True and false pelvis is separated by:
   a) Inferior rami of pubis
   b) Ischial tuberosity
   c) Iliopectineal line
   d) Both a and b
   e) Ischial tuberosity

   Answer: c

The iliopectineal line runs forwards from the apex of the auricular surface and clearly demarcates the true from the false pelvis. The interior pole of the ischial bone bears the **ischial tuberosity.** This is easily palpated through the buttock when the hip is flexed and it is this on which you sit.

-The pelvis tilts forwards in the erect posture so that the plane of its inlet is at an angle, of 60 degrees to the horizontal. To place the articulated pelvis in the position it adopts in standing, **position it against a wall** so that the anterior superior iliac spine and the top of the body of the pubis touch it.

10. Sacral hiatus transmits:
    a) S4
    b) S5
    c) S1
    d) S2
    e) All of above
       Answer: b

11. Sure sign for sacral hiatus is:
    a) Sacral cornu
    b) Sacral promontory
    c) C7 spine
    d) Ischial tuberosity
    e) Ischial spine
       Answer: a

12. False statement among following is:
    a) Fusion of fifth lumber vertebrae with sacrum is called lumberization of sacral vertebrae
    b) Separation of first sacral vertebrae from rest of sacrum is called lumberization of sacral vertebrae
    c) Dural sheath terminate at level of S2
    d) Coccyx is made up of 5 diminitive vertebrae
    e) Symphysis pubis is cartilaginous joint
       Answer: a

• Inferiorly, the canal terminates at the sacral hiatus, which faces posteriorly and transmits the fifth sacral nerve. The lower extremity of the hiatus bears a **sacral cornu** on either side, which can be easily palpated with the finger immediately above the natal cleft. This is a sure guide to the canal when performing a **sacral block**.
•The fifth lumbar vertebra may occasionally fuse partly or wholly with the sacrum ('sacralization of L5'). The first

segment of the sacrum may be partly or completely separate from the rest of the bone ('lumbarization of S1'). ● The **dural sheath terminates** distally at the level of the **second piece** of the sacrum. This level corresponds to the level of the **sacral dimple** on either side. Below this level, the sacral canal is filled with the loose connective tissue of the extradural space, the lower filaments of the cauda equine, and the filum terminale. The extradural space can be entered through the sacral hiatus to perform an extradural anaesthetic block .

The coccyx

The coccyx (figure 2.4) is made up of three to five diminutive vertebrae and articulates with the lower end of the sacrum.

Joints and ligaments of the pelvis

The *symphysis pubis* is the cartilaginous joint between the body of the pubis on either side. It is strengthened by fibrous ligaments, especially above and below.

13. Most powerfull ligament in body is:
    a) Anterior sacroiliac ligament
    b) Posterior sacroiliac ligament
    c) Sacrotuberous ligament
    d) Sacrospinous ligament
    e) Anterior cruciate ligament
    Answer: b

The *sacroiliac joint* is a synovial joint , the sacrum hangs like a wedge between these two joints and is supported by the *posterior sacroiliac ligament* on each side. Since these support the whole weight of the body, it is not surprising that they are the most powerful ligaments in the body.

In addition, there are the *sacrotuberous* and the *sacrospinous ligaments* , which define two exits from the pelvis:

1. The *greater sciatic foramen* — between the greater sciatic notch and the sacrospinous ligament.

2. The *lesser sciatic foramen* — between the lesser sciatic notch and the sacrospinous and sacrotuberous ligaments.

14. Which of following is not difference between male and female pelvis visible on x –ray:

a) Heart shaped in male and oval in female
b) Pubic angle is narrow in male and wide in female
c) Soft tissue shadow scrotum is seen in female
d) Anteroposterior diameter is more in female
e) Sacrum is wide in female
Answer: c

15. Which of following indicate pelvis is contracted:
a) Diagonal conjugate 12.5 cm
b) Sacral promontory can be easily reached
c) Transvers diameter 13 cm
d) Clinched fist should fit between ischial tuberosities
e) Pelvic walls concave
Answer: b

Differences which are obvious when looking at an x-ray of the pelvis between male and female are:
-The pelvic inlet is heart-shaped in the male and comparatively larger and oval in the female. The inlet is enlarged in the female because the ala of the sacrum on either side is as wide as the transverse width of the body of the sacrum. In the male, each ala is only about half the width of the body.
-A very constant difference is that the angle between the inferior pubic rami is narrow in the male and wide in the female — thus, of course, widening the bony pelvic outlet.* In the male it corresponds to the angle formed between the index and the middle finger, whereas in the female it corresponds to the angle formed between the outstretched thumb and index finger.
-*The transverse diameter of the outlet* of the pelvis is assessed clinically by measuring the distance between the ischial tuberosities in a plane passing across the anal orifice.
-The *anteroposterior diameter of the outlet* is measured from the inferior aspect of the pubic symphysis to the coccyx.
-The most useful measurement is the *diagonal conjugate*: the distance between the lower margin of the pubic symphysis to the promontory of the sacrum. 12.5 cm. It is not possible, in the normal pelvis, to reach the sacral promontory on vaginal examination — if it is possible, the pelvis is seriously contracted.

Obstetrical pelvic measurements

	transverse	oblique	anteroposterior
Inlet	12.5 cm	11.5 cm	10 cm
Mid pelvis	11.5 cm	11.5 cm	11.5 cm
Outlet	10 cm	11.5 cm	12.5 cm

Comparison of male and female pelvis

	male	female
General structure	heavy and thick	light and thin
Joint surfaces	large	small
Muscle attachments	well marked	rather indistinct
False pelvis	deep	shallow
Pelvic inlet	heart-shaped	oval
Pelvic canal	long and tapered	short with almost parallel sides
Pelvic outlet	small	large
Subpubic angle (between Inferior pubic rami)	narrow	wide(>90)
Acetabulum	large	small
Ischial tuberosities	inturned	everted
Obturator foramen	round	oval

16. Levator ani is supplied by:
    a) Pudendal nerve
    b) Obturator nerve
    c) Femoral nerve
    d) Hypogastric nerve
    e) Sciatic verve
    Answer: a

Levator ani
- This is a broad, thin muscle.
- It arises from the posterior aspect of the body of the Pubis, from the ischial spine, and from the dense fascia Covering obturator internus between these two attachments.
- The fibres pass medially and downwards to meet the Muscle of the opposite side in a raphe.

• The anterior fibres pass backwards to loop around the posterior aspect of the vagina to meet in the fi brous perineal body.

• The middle fibres pass backwards and downwards around the posterior aspect of the terminal part of the rectum to the fibrous anococcygeal body and blend with the anal sphincter muscles.

• The posterior fibres pass to attach to the coccyx and to a midline raphe between the coccyx and the anococcygeal body. Levator ani provides muscular support to the pelvic
Viscera, especially when intra-abdominal pressure is
Raised in micturition, defecation, and parturition.

• Its innermost fibres, often termed the *puborectalis* , form a sling around the anorectal junction. This maintains the sharp angulation between the rectum and the anal canal, which can be appreciated on rectal examination and on sigmoidoscopy.

• Levator ani is supplied by the pudendal nerve.

17. Which of following is not containt of superfascial perineal pouch :

a) Ischiocavernosus muscle
b) Bulbospongiosus muscle
c) Superficial transverse perineal muscle
d) Deep transverse perineal muscle
e) Crura of clotoris

Answer: d

Superficial to the perineal membrane is the *superficial perineal pouch* . The
Contents of this pouch include:

• Ischiocavernosus muscle
• Bulbospongiosus muscle
• Superficialtransverse perineal muscle
• Crura of the clitoris (crura of the penis in the male)
• Vestibular bulbs (bulb of the penis in the male)
• The greater vestibular glands (Bartholin's).

18. False statement about anal triangle is:

a) Medially levator ani and external anal sphincter
b) Fascia over obturator internus with Alcock`s canal

c) Roof levator ani

d) Floor skin and fat

e) Posteriorly urogenital perineum

Answer: e

This triangle lies between the ischial tuberosity on each side of the coccyx. It is roofed by levator ani, and contains the anal canal with its encircling sphincters and with the ischioanal fossa on either side. The *ischioanal fossa* is of surgical importance because of the frequency with which it may become infected and because the pudendal nerve and vessels lie in its lateral wall.

Its boundaries are:

● Medially — the fascia over the inferior aspect of the Levator ani and the external anal sphincter.

● Laterally — the fascia over obturator internus on the inner side wall of the pelvis. Contained within a tunnel **(the pudendal or Alcock's canal) in the fascia covering this muscle are the pudendal nerve (S2,S3, and S4) and the internal pudendal artery and vein**. These give off the inferior rectal vessels and nerve, supplying the external anal sphincter and perianal skin, and then pass forward to supply the perineal tissues.

● Anteriorly — the urogenital perineum.

● **Posteriorly — the sacrotuberous ligament, covered behind by gluteus maximum.**

● Floor — skin and subcutaneous fat.

● Contents — fat.

19. Which of following is not true support of uterus:

a) Uterosacral ligament

b) Broad ligament

c) Cardinal ligament

d) Levator ani

e) Pubocervical ligament

Answer: b

20. Uterus pierce:

a) Uterosacral ligament

b) Broad ligament

c) Cardinal ligament

d) Levator ani

e) Pubocervical ligament

Answer: c

21. Canal of nuck present in:

a) Labia majora

b) Labia minora

c) Inguinal canal

d) Obturator fossa

e) Femoral canal

Answer: a

The pelvic fascia is the connective tissue that covers the pelvic walls and the viscera lying within the pelvic cavity. It is divided into the parietal and the endopelvic fascia. The *parietal fascia* covers the walls and the floor of the pelvic cavity. It is thickened over obturator internus, where it gives attachment to levator ani. The spinal nerves lie outside this fascia, while the pelvic vessels lie internal to it. The *endopelvic fascia* is the extraperitoneal connective tissue that covers

The uterus (the parametrium), vagina, bladder, and rectum. Three condensations of the connective tissue sling the pelvic organs from the walls of the pelvis **1.** The *cardinal ligaments* (also known as the transverse cervical or Mackenrodt's ligaments) pass laterally on each side from the cervix and upper vagina to the side wall of the pelvis. They are made up of fibrous connective tissue with some involuntary muscle and are pierced in their upper part by the ureter on each side.

The *pubocervical fascia* extends forward on either side of the bladder from the lateral part of the cardinal ligament on each side of the pubis, acting as a sling for the bladder. The *uterosacral ligaments* pass backwards on either side from the posterolateral aspect of the cervix at the level of its isthmus, and from the lateral fornix of the vagina in the lateral boundary of the pouch of douglas. They attach to the periosteum in front of the sacroiliac joint and lateral part of the third piece of the sacrum.

These ligaments, in conjunction with levator ani, act as supports to the uterine cervix and the vaginal vault. In uterine prolapse these ligaments are stretched.

Two other ligaments take attachment from the uterus:

1.The *broad ligament* is a fold of peritoneum on either side that connects the lateral margin of the body of the uterus to the side wall of the pelvis on either side . The uterus and its broad ligaments thus form a transverse partition across the pelvis, which defines an anterior compartment, the *uterovesical pouch* , containing the bladder, and a posterior compartment, the *recto-uterine pouch* or *pouch of douglas* , which contains the rectum.

The broad ligament contains or carries:

• The uterine tube in its free edge
• The ovary, attached by its mesovarium to its posterior aspect
• The round ligament on its anterior aspect
• The ovarian ligament crossing from the ovary to the Cornu of the uterus
• Uterine vessels, branches of the ovarian vessels,

Lymphatics, and autonomic nerves.

The ureter passes forwards to the bladder deep to the broad ligament and lateral to, and immediately above, The lateral fornix of the vagina

2.The *round ligament* , which is a fibromuscular cord, passes from the lateral angle of the uterus in the anterior layer of the broad ligament to the internal inguinal ring. It then transverses the inguinal canal to the labium majus.

Note that the round ligament, taken with the ovarian ligament, is the female equivalent of the male gubernaculum testis, along which the fetal testis descends to the scrotum.

Patent processus vaginalis around round ligament form canal of nuck in labia majora

22. Wrong statement among following is:

    a) Cervix project into anterior vaginal wall

    b) Posterior vaginal wall is 10cm

    c) Anterior to vagina is pouch of Douglas

    d) Posterior to vagina is rectum and anal canal

    e) Lateraly ureter and levator ani

Answer: c

The cervix projects into the anterior part of the vault of the vagina, so that the continuous gutter that surrounds the cervix is shallow anteriorly, where the vaginal wall is some **7.5** cm in length, and deep posteriorly, where the wall is about 10 cm long. This continuous gutter is divided, for convenience of description, into the anterior, posterior, and lateral *fornices* (fornix = arch).

Relations

• the vagina is related anteriorly to the cervix above, then to the base of the bladder, and then to the urethra. The urethra is firmly embedded in the vaginal wall, opening in front of the vaginal orifice into the vestibule.

• the posterior fornix and the upper 2 cm of the posterior wall of the vagina is covered by the peritoneum of the recto-uterine pouch — the pouch of douglas — and comes into contact, usually, with loops of small intestine. It is here, of course, that collections of fluid such as blood or pus may be detected on bimanual vaginal examination. Below the pouch, the posterior vaginal wall lies against the anterior aspect of the rectum and then the anal canal, separated by the perineal body.

• laterally — the levator ani, the pelvic fascia, and the ureter on each side, lying immediately above the lateral fornix — indeed, rarely an impacted ureteric calculus can be palpated at this side on vaginal examination!

The *arterial supply* of the vagina derives from the vaginal, uterine, internal pudendal, and middle rectal branches of the internal iliac artery, while a venous plexus drains via the vaginal vein into the internal iliac vein.

Lymphatic drainage **can be considered in**
Thirds:

Upper third — to the external and internal iliac nodes
Middle third — to the internal iliac nodes
Lower third — to the inguinal nodes

23. False statement about uterus is:
    a) In nulliparous women external Os is circular
    b) In pregnancy cervix has consistency like nose
    c) Child cervix is twice size of body of uterus
    d) Isthmus is 1.5cm in length

    e) In anteverted uterus anterior lip of cervix first felt
      Answer: b

• The isthmus is 1.5 cm in length. Its junction with the uterine body is marked by the internal os within the uterine cavity. It is the isthmus that becomes the lower segment of the uterus in pregnancy.

• In the nulliparous female the external os is circular, but it becomes a transverse slit, with an anterior and a posterior lip, after childbirth.

• The non-pregnant cervix is firm, with the consistency of the tip of the nose. In pregnancy it softens, and has the consistency of the lips.

• The fetal cervix is considerably larger than the body of the uterus. In the child the cervix is twice the size of the body (the infantile uterus). During puberty, the uterus enlarges, by relative overgrowth of its body, to reach adult size and proportions.

• in the adult, the uterus bends forward on itself at the Level of the internal os — anteflexion of the uterus — while the cervix tips posteriorly with the axis of the vagina at roughly a right-angle — anteversion of the uterus. Thus, the uterus comes to lie in almost a horizontal plane

• In *retroflexion of the uterus* the axis of the body passes upwards and backwards in relation to the axis of the cervix. In *retroversion of the uterus* the axis of the cervix passes upwards and backwards

• In normal vaginal examination the anterior lip of the cervix is the lowermost part to be felt, while in retroversion posterior lip of cervix first to felt.

    24.. False statement about uterus is:
      a) Anteriorly uterovesical pouch of peritoneum
      b) Ureter is situated 12 mm lateral to lateral vaginal fornix
      c) Peritoneum covers whole of uterus
      d) Uterine artery is a branch of internal iliac artery and it is lies above ureter and supply uterus at level of isthmus
      e) Ovarian artery is a branch of aorta
        Answer: c

• Anteriorly the uterine body relates to the uterovesical Pouch of peritoneum

• posteriorly lies the recto-uterine pouch (pouch of Douglas), • laterally lies the broad ligament and its contents — The uterine tube, ovary, blood vessels, lymphatics, and Autonomic nerves. The ureter passes below the broad Ligament and uterine vessels and is situated 12 mm Lateral to the supravaginal cervix, immediately above the lateral vaginal fornix. It is here that the ureter may be accidentally damaged, divided, or tied when the uterine vessels are clamped during a hysterectomy.

Peritoneal relationships

The body of the uterus is covered with peritoneum of the pelvic floor except where it is reflected off at two sites —

Laterally at the broad ligament on either side and anteriorly onto the bladder at the level of the uterus isthmus.

Anteriorly the peritoneum is only loosely adherent, to allow for bladder distension. Posteriorly the peritoneum continues.

Inferiorly to cover the posterior wall of the upper quarter of the vagina, so that on vaginal examination, a finger in the posterior fornix of the vagina is only about 1 mm away from the peritoneum of the pelvic floor.

Blood supply

The principal arterial supply is from the uterine artery, a branch of the internal iliac artery.

25. Lymphatic drainage of uterus and fallopian tube is:
    a) Fundus to inguinal lymph node and para-aortic lymph node
    b) Body of uterus to external iliac group of lymph node
    c) Cervix external iliac, internal iliac and sacral group of lymph node
    d) Fallopian tube and ovarian lymphatic passes to para-aortic lymph node
    e) All of above

    Answer: e

Lymphatic drainage of uterus:

• The fundus, together with the uterine tubes and the Ovaries along the ovarian vessels to the paraaortic lymph nodes and along the round ligament to inguinal lymph nodes.

• The body of the uterus: along the broad ligament To nodes lying along the external iliac blood vessels.

• The cervix drains in three directions: laterally, in the Broad ligament, to the **external iliac nodes**; posterolaterally along the uterine vessels to the **internal iliac nodes;** and posteriorly along the recto-uterine fold to the **sacral lymph nodes.**

The uterine (fallopian) tubes

10 cm in length

Made up of four parts:

1. *The infundibulum*

2. *The ampulla*

3. *The isthmus*

4. *The interstitial part*

It is lined throuGHout by a **ciliated columnar**

Epithelium.

Blood supply: laterally by the ovarian artery and vein and medially by the uterine vessels.

Lymphatic drainage links with that of the ovary and passes to the para-aortic nodes.

26. False statement about ovary is:
    a) Ovary is almond shape organ with diameter of 4 cm
    b) External iliac vessel present in anterior relation of ovarian fossa
    c) Ovarian fossa contain perineal nerve
    d) Right ovarian vein drain into inferior vena cava
    e) Left ovarian vein drain into left renal vein
       Answer: c

27. False statement about ovary is:
    a) Ovary is almond shape organ with diameter of 4 cm
    b) External iliac vessel present in anterior relation of ovarian fossa
    c) Ovarian fossa contain obturator nerve
    d) Right ovarian vein drain into right ovarian vein
    e) Left ovarian vein drain into left renal vein

Answer: d

28. False statement about ovary is:
    a) Ovary is almond shape organ with diameter of 4 cm
    b) External iliac vessel present in posterior relation of ovarian fossa
    c) Ovarian fossa contain obturator nerve
    d) Right ovarian vein drain into inferior vena cava
    e) Left ovarian vein drain into left renal vein
    Answer: b

The ovary is an almond-shaped organ 4 cm in length. Attach to back of broad ligament by *mesovarium* .

Two ligaments of ovary are:

-infundibulopelvic ligament (sometimes called the suspensory ligament of the ovary), in which pass the ovarian vessels, lymphatics, and autonomic nerves from the side wall of the pelvis, and ovarian ligament, which passes to the cornu of the Uterus.

Ovarian fossa:

On the side wall of the pelvis.

Present in depression between the external iliac vessels anteriorly, and the internal iliac vessels together with the ureter posteriorly; it contains the obturator nerve.

Blood supply

The ovarian artery arises from the aorta just below the level of the renal artery. The ovarian vein drains, on the right, into the inferior vena cava at the same level, while on the left it opens into the left renal vein.

Lymphatics pass to the para-aorta nodes at the level of the renal vessels.

Autonomic nerve supply : T 10

29. Term vulva include:
    a) Mons pubis
    b) Labia majora and minora
    c) Clitoris
    d) Grater vestubular gland
    e) All of above
    Answer: e

The external genitalia in the female comprise the mons pubis, the labia majora and minora, the vestibule of the Vagina, the clitoris, the bulb of the vestibule, and the greater vestibular (Bartholin) glands. The general term *vulva* (or pudendum) includes all these structures.

30. True statement among following is:
    a) Mons pubis is made up of adipose tissue and cover with hair and sebaceous gland
    b) Cleft between labia majora is termed as vestibule
    c) Ischiocavernosus muscle cut during medio-lateral episiotomy
    d) Clitoris contain pair of carpora cavernosa
    e) Bulb of vestibule lies on each side of ischiocavernosus muscle
    Answer: a

31. Space between labia minora called:
    a) Vulva
    b) Vestibule
    c) Perineum
    d) Mons pubis
    e) Bulb of vestibule
    Answer: b

The mons pubis

This rounded eminence anterior to the pubic symphysis is formed by subcutaneous adipose tissue. At puberty it becomes covered with hair that has a horizontal upper limit, in contrast to the male, where the pubic hair extends upwards towards the umbilicus in and adjacent to the median line.

The labia majora and minora

The labia major are two folds of skin that meet anteriorly at the mons and posteriorly in the midline anterior to the anal orifice. They are more obvious anteriorly. The midline cleft between the **labia majora is termed the *vulval cleft*.** Within the cleft lie the thin, vascular folds of skin, the **labia minora, which lack both hair and sebaceous glands**. The space between these folds is termed *the vestibule*, into which opens the urethral orifice, 2.5 cm behind the clitoris, and behind the urethra lies the opening of the vagina. The *bulbospongiosus muscle* runs on either side from its attachment to the perineal body in front of the anal canal beneath the skin of the vestibule to insert into the clitoris. Laterally, the *ischiocavernosus muscle* runs from the medial surface of the ramus of the ischium forward and medially to insert into the clitoris. The *superficial transverse perineal muscles* run laterally from the perineal body to the ischial ramus .

The clitoris

This is the female equivalent of the penis,it consists, like the penis, of three columns of erectile tissue but, unlike the penis, of course, it does not transmit the urethra, which opens behind it.

• the erectile tissue comprises the corpora cavernosa and the bulbs of the vestibule. The paired *corpora cavernosa* lie deep to the ischiocavernosus muscle and arise from the ischiopubic ramus on each side. They meet in the body of the clitoris. The paired *bulbs of the vestibule* lie on each side deep to the bulbospongiosus muscle. Anteriorly each continues as a thin band of erectile tissue into the clitoris, uniting into a strand that expands into the *glans* at its tip. The bulbs of the vestibule, together with the glans of the clitoris, are equivalent to the corpus spongiosum and glans of the male. The anterior ends of the labia Minora split to surround the clitoris, providing it with a Prepuce.

32. Grater vestibular gland open at
   a) Posterior part of cervix
   b) Lateral wall of vagina at introitus
   c) Groove between vaginal orifice and posterior part of labia minora
   d) Anterior part of vagina
   e) Near urethral opening
   Answer: c

The greater vestibular glands of bartholin

These comprise a pair of lobulated, pea-shaped, mucus secreting glands that lie deep to the posterior parts of the labia majora. They are impalpable when healthy but become obvious when inflamed or distended. Each drains by a 2.5 cm-long duct, which opens into the groove between the vaginal orifice and the posterior part of the labium minus.

Anteriorly each gland is overlapped superficially by the vestibular bulb.

33. Branches of internal pudendal artery are:
   a) Posterior labial branch

b) Artery to bulb of vestibule
c) Dorsal artery of clitoris
d) Deep artery of clitoris
e) All of above
   Answer: e

Blood supply of external genatalia:
Internal pudendal artery and vein branch of internal iliac vessels and run forward on the lateral wall of the ischioanal fossa in Alcock's canal.
These vessels are:
● Posterior labial branches
● The artery and vein of the bulb
● The deep vessels of the clitoris
● The dorsal vessels of the clitoris
These branches of the internal pudendal vessels anastomose with terminal branches of the superficial external pudendal vessels of the femoral artery and vein.

34. Medial part of labia majora is supplied by:
   a) Ilioinguinal nerve
   b) Genitofemoral nerve
   c) Pudendal nerve
   d) Iliohypogastric nerve
   e) Obturator nerve
      Answer: c

Nerve supply of exernal genitalia
The skin of the mons pubis and the adjacent anterolateral parts of the labia majora : spinal segment L1 through the *ilioinguinal* and *genitofemoral nerves*. The rest of the external genitalia: S3 via the *pudendal*
Nerve via its perineal branch.

35. Which of following structure not develop from mesonephric duct:
   a) Vas deference
   b) Epoophoron and mesoophoron
   c) Duct of gartner
   d) Prostatic utricle
   e) Epididymis
      Answer: d

36. Which of following structure not develop from paramesonephric duct:
    a) Appendix of testes
    b) Prostatic utricle
    c) Duct of Gartner
    d) Fallopian tube
    e) Upper third of vagina
       Answer: c

37. Uterine muscle develops from:
    a) Endoderm
    b) Ectoderm
    c) Mesoderm
    d) Neural crest
    e) All of above
       Answer: c

Embryology of the genital tract
• In the male the paramesonephric duct disappears,
Apart from the appendix testis (a tiny cystic structure perched on the upper pole of the testis, which may undergo torsion) and the prostatic utricle (a short sinus leading into the posterior aspect of the prostatic Urethra).
• In the female the mesonephric duct system, which in the male develops into the epididymis and the vas deferens, persists only as small cystic remnants alongside the genital tract termed the epoophoron, mesoophoron, and the ducts of gartner.
• in the female the paramesonephric ducts cranially become the fallopian tubes. More caudally, they sweep together and fuse in the midline to become the epithelium of the body of the uterus, the cervix, and the upper third of the vagina — at first a solid cord that then canalizes.
The rest of the vaginal epithelium forms by canalization of the solid sinuvaginal node at the back of the Urogenital sinus. (this accounts for the difference in the lymphatic drainage of the upper and lower vagina.)
• the musculature of the genital tract derives from the surrounding mesoderm, so that the cystic remnants of the mesonephric ducts in the female are found embedded in the myometrium, the cervix, and the wall of the vagina.

• as the paramesonephric ducts sweep together and
Fuse in their distal parts, they drag a peritoneal fold with them on either side — this becomes the broad ligament.

38. Round ligament develops from:
   a) Germinal ridge
   b) Upper part of gubernaculum
   c) Lower part of gubernaculum
   d) Ectoderm
   e) Sino vaginal bulb
      Answer: c

Both the ovary and the testis develop from a germinal ridge medial to the mesonephros at about the level of the first lumbar vertebra.
-*gubernaculum:* along this strand testis in the male descends into the scrotum. The ovary too descends, dragging its blood supply, lymphatics, and nerve supply with it, but it impacts against the posterior aspect of the broad ligament. The gubernaculum
Persists as the *ovarian ligament*, which passes from the ovary across the posterior aspect of the broad ligament to the side of the uterus and, from there, as the *round ligament*, passing across the front of the broad ligament to the side wall of the pelvis to traverse the inguinal canal and end in the labium majus.

39. Extravasated urine does not go into:
   a) Superfascial perineal pouch
   b) Thigh
   c) Dartos fascia of scrotum
   d) Scarpa`s fascia of anterior abdominal wall
   e) None of above
      Answer: b

The cavernous erectile tissues (the crura and the bulb), their surrounding skeletal muscles (ischiocavernosus and bulbospongiosus respectively), and the superficial transverse perineal muscles are all covered by colles fascia, to create the superficial perineal pouch or space. Colles fascia is continuous with dartos fascia of the scrotum and scarpa's fascia of the anterior abdominal wall, but does not extend into the thigh, hence extravasated urine does not go into the thigh.

40. Puckering of breast tissue because of
   a) Cowper`s ligament
   b) Scarpa`s fascia
   c) Fascia of camphor
   d) Pectoralis major
   e) None of above
      Answer: a

The skin is connected to the deep fascia by suspensory ligaments of the breast (Cowper's Ligament), which are responsible for skin 'puckering' In breast disease.

Important questins:

1. Fallopian tube is lined by:
   A) simple squamous
   B) simple cuboidal
   C) simple columnar
   D) stratified squamous
   E) stratified cuboidal
   Answer : c

2. Vagina is lined by:
   A) Simple squamous
   B) Simple cuboidal
   C) Simple columnar
   D) Stratified squamous
   E) Stratified cuboidal
   Answer: d

3. Urinary bladder is lined by:
   A) Simple squamous
   B) Simple cuboidal
   C) Stratified transitional
   D) Stratified squamous
   E) Stratified cuboidal

Answer: c

4. Somatic nervous system do not cross midline. Its posterior primary ramus supply:
   A) Erector spinae and overlying skin
   B) Cervical plexus
   C) Brachial plexus
   D) Lumber plexus
   E) Sacral plexus
   Answer: a

5. Preganglionic autonomic fibers are
   A) Mylinated
   B) Unmylinated
   C) ACH is neurotransmitter at ganglion
   D) Both a and c
   E) Both band c
   Answer: d

6. Which of the following is not sympathetic effect:
   A) Iincrease heart rate
   B) Constriction of coronary artery
   C) Dilates bronchial tree
   D) Relaxes detrusor muscle
   E) Constrict smooth muscle sphincter
   Answer: b

7. Which of the following is parasympathetic effect:
   A) Increase peristalsis
   B) Constriction of coronary artery
   C) Dilates bronchial tree
   D) Relaxes detrusor muscle
   E) Constrict smooth muscle sphincter
   Answer: a

8. Dura mater end at S2, epidural space is situated between:
   A) Dura mater and spinal canal
   B) Dura mater and arachnoid mater
   C) Arachnoid mater and pia mater
   D) Pia mater and spinal cord

E) None of above

Answer: a

9. Touch and vibration transmitted by

A) Lateral spinothalamic tract

B) Anterior spinothalamic tract

C) Posterior columns

D) Lateral spinocerebellar tract

E) Anterior cerebro spinal tract

Answer c

10. Acidophilic cells produce :

A) ACTH

B) FSH

C) TSH

D) GH

E) LH

Answer: d

11. Cisterna chyli lies over

A) L1,L2

B) T12,L1

C) L2,L3

D) L4,L5

E) T11,T12

Answer: a

12. Clitoris drain into :

A) Superficial inguinal lymph node

B) Deep inguinal lymph node

C) External iliac nodes

D) Internal iliac nodes

E) Obturator nodes

Answer b

13. Vulva drain into

A) Superficial inguinal lymph node

B) Deep inguinal lymph node

C) External iliac nodes

D) Internal iliac nodes

E) Deep femoral lymph node of cloquet

Answer e

14. Cervix and upper one third of vagina drain into:

A) Superficial inguinal lymph node

B) Deep inguinal lymph node

C) External iliac nodes

D) Internal iliac nodes

E) Obturator nodes

Answer d

15. Oxygenated blood from umbilical vein to inferior vena cava is bypasses by:

A) Ductus venosus

B) Foramen ovale

C) Dctus arteriosus

D) Ligamentum arteriosum

E) Ligamentum venosum

Answer: a

16. Ductus venosus become:

A) Medial umbilical ligament

B) Foramen ovale

C) Ductus arteriosus

D) Ligamentum arteriosum

E) Ligamentum venosum

Answer: e

17. Obliterated remains of Urachus called:

A) Median umbilical ligament

B) Medial umbilical ligament

C) Ductus arteriosus

D) Ligamentum arteriosum

E) Ligamentum venosum

Answer: a

18. Aorta enters abdomen at:

A) L1

B) L2

C) L3

D) L4

E) T12

Answer: e

19. Coeliac artery a ventral branch of aorta arises at

A) L1

B) L2

C) L3

D) L4

E) T12

Answer: a

20. Superior mesenteric artery a ventral branch of aorta arises at

A) L1

B) L2

C) L3

D) L4

E) T12

Answer: b

21. Inferior mesenteric artery a ventral branch of aorta arises at

A) L1

B) L2

C) L3

D) L4

E) T12

Answer: c

22. Aorta arises divide into right and left common iliac artery at:

A) L1

B) L2

C) L3

D) L4

E) T12

Answer: d

23. Terminal branches of aorta is
    A) Right and left common iliac artery
    B) Median sacral artery
    C) Phrenic artery, suprarenal artery,
    D) Renal artery and gonadal artery
    E) Both a and b
    Answer: e

24. Common iliac artery divides into internal and external iliac artery at
    A) L1
    B) L2
    C) L3
    D) L4
    E) Sacroiliac joint
    Answer: e

25. External ilia artery become femoral artery beyond
    A) L1
    B) L2
    C) L3
    D) Inguinal ligament
    E) Sacroiliac joint
    Answer: d

26. Common iliac vein join to form IVC behind right iliac vein at :
    A) L1
    B) L2
    C) L3
    D) L4
    E) L5
    Answer: e

27. IVC pierces diaphragm at level of :
    a) L1
    B) L2
    C) T12
    D) T10

E) T8

Answer: e

28. Spread of malignancy from pelvic viscera to vertebral venous plexus system via:
    a) Lateral sacral vessels
    b) Lumbar vein
    c) Posterior intercostal
    d) Vertebral vein
    e) Inferior mesenteric vein
       Answer: a

29. Obstetric conjugate is:

    a) 10.5cm

    b) 12cm

    c) 13cm

    d) 15cm

    e) 17cm

Answer: a

30. Vitamin d deficiency cause:
    A) Rachitic pelvis
    B) Android pelvis
    C) Anthropoid pelvis
    D) Platypelloid pelvis
    E) Gynaecoid pelvis
    Answer: a

31. Presenting diameter of fetal skull is smallest with following presentation:
    A) Occipital presentation
    B) Face presentation
    C) Vertex presentation
    D) Brow presentation

E) Both a and b

Answer: e

32. Angle of Louis lies at the level of :

A) T1

B) T2

C) T3

D) T4

E) T5

Answer: d

33. True ribs present:

A) 1 to 7

B) 8 to 10

C) 11 to 12

D) 1 to 8

E) 8 to 12

Answer: a

34. Aspiration or insertion of chest drain is usually done through:

A) Mid clavicular line 5th intercostal space by running needle or drain over the rib

B) Mid axillary line 5th intercostal space by running needle or drain over the rib

C) Mid clavicular line 5th intercostal space by running needle or drain under the rib

D) Mid axillar line 5th intercostal space by running needle or drain under the rib

E) Mid clavicular line 4th intercostal space by running needle or drain over the rib

Answer: b

35. Oesophageal opening in the diaphragm usually present at the level of :

A) T12

B) T8

C) T11

D) T10

E) T9

Answer: d

36. Inferior vena caval opening in the diaphragm usually present at the level of :

A) T12

B) T8

C) T11

D) T10

E) T9

Answer: b

37. Aortic opening in the diaphragm usually present at the level of :

A) T12

B) T8

C) T11

D) T10

E) T9

Answer:a

38. Transpyloric plane is usually present hand breath below xiphod process , at ninth coastal cartilage, marks termination of spinal cord is correspond to vertebral level:

A) T12

B) L1

C) T11

D) T10

E) T9

Answer: b

39. Transpyloric level indicates:

A) Pylorus of stomach

B) Duodenojejunal flexure

C) Fundus of gall bladder

D) Renal hila and neck of pancreas

E) All of the above

Answer: d

40. Bifurcation of abdominal aorta present at level of plane of iliac crests which is at level of :

A) T12

B) L3

C) L4

D) T10

E) T8

Answer: c

41. In order to avoid injury to inferior epigastric vessel needle for paracentesis must pass through:

A) Lateral to mc Burney`s point

B) Medial to mc Burney`s point

C) Medial to Palmer`s point

D) Lateral to Palmer`s point

E) Umbilicus

Answer: a

42. Pyramidalis is supplied by:

A) Subcostal nerve

B) T8

C) T11

D) T10

E) T9

Answer: a

43. Deep inguinal ring which is defect in fascia transversalis, is lies at:

A) Mid-inguinal canal point

B) Mid point of inguinal ligament

C) Divergent fibres of external oblique

D) Heselbach triangle

E) Femoral ring

Answer: b

44. Which of the following is not component of spermatic cord :

A) Vas deferens

B) Genital branch of genitofemoral nerve

C) Cremasteric artery

D) Inferior epigastric artery

E) Pampiniform venous plexous

Answer: d

45. Wrong statement regarding femoral sheath is :

A) Femoral nerve lies in sheath

B) Femoral artery lies in sheath

C) Femoral vein lies in sheath

D) Femoral canal lies in sheath

E) Lacunar ligament lies medialy

Answer: a

46. Wrong statement regarding epiploic foramen is:

A) Superiorly caudate lobe of liver

B) Inferiorly first part of duodenum

C) Posteriorly inferior vena cava,

D) Anteriorly portal vein, hepatic artery, common bile duct

E) Left adrenal gland posteriorly

Answer: e

47. True statement among following is:

A) Superior pancreaticoduodenal artery is branch of superior mesenteric artery.

B) Inferior mesenteric artery is a branch of superior mesenteric artery

C) Superior mesenteric artery passes over superior to third part of duodenum

D) Inferior mesenteric artery terminate as middle rectal artery

E) Splenic artery give right gastro epiploic artery

Answer: b

48. Which of the following is false related to acute appendicitis in preganancy:

A) Signs can be relatively subtle

B) Progression of pathology can be rapid due to failure of omentum to access problem and seal it off

C) Upward displacement of caecum

D) Surgical incision of appendicectomy at mc Burney`s point

E) Non of above

Answer: d

49. Right renal artery passes behind:

A) Diaphragm

B) Inferior vena cava

C) Aorta

D) Psoas muscle

E) Ureter

Answer: b

50. False statement among following is:

A) Right ovarian artery crosses inferior vena cava and is crossed by terminal ileal vein, caecal vein, ileocolic vein

B) Right vein drain into right renal vein

C) Left common iliac artery is crossed by superior mesenteric vessels

D) Inferior epigastric artery and circumflex iliac artery arises just above inguinal ligament

E) Genitofemoral nerve lies anterior to psoas muscle

Answer: b

51. 35 year old patient complain of pain in knee jont. USG 1 month back suggestive of ovarian cyst. What can be cause of pain in knee joint:

A) Obturator nerve irritation

B) Lateral cutaneous nerve of thigh irritation

C) Femoral nerve irritation

D) Sacral nerve irritation

E) Genitofemoral nerve irritation

Answer: a

52. Which of the following is not branch of internal iliac artery:

A) Uterine artery

B) Ovarian artery

C) Inferior gluteal artery

D)Middle rectal artery

E) Internal pudendal artery

Answer: b

53.Pudendal nerve arises from

A) S2 to S4

B) S1 to S5

C) L4, L5,S1

D) L5 S1-2

E) S4

Answer: a

54.Which of the following is not contain of superficial perineal pouch

A) Bulbospongiosus muscle

B) Ischiocavernosus muscle

C) Superficial transverse perineal muscle

D) External urethral sphincter

E) Corpus spongiosum

Answer: d

55.False statement among following about ischiorectal fossa is :

A) Posteriorly, the sacrotuberous ligament and gluteus maximus muscle

B) Medially fascia over levator ani and external anal sphincter

C) Laterally ischial tuberosity with obturator internus muscle

D) Pudendal (alcock) canal medially

E) Posteriorly, perineal branch of S4 and perforating cutaneous branch

Answer: d

56.Pudendal nerve block is given by piercing needle just beyond ischial spine. Good test of efficacy is

A) Loss of anal reflex

B) Relaxation of pelvic floor

C) Loss of sensation of vulva

D) Loss of sensation of lower third of vagina

E) All of the above

Answer: e

57. Pelvic peritoneum is supplied by:

A) Perineal branch of S4

B) Obturator nerve(L2-4)

C) Pudendal nerve

D) Nerve to obturator internus

E) Sciatic nerve

Answer: b

58. False statement regarding boundaries of ovarian fossa

A) Obturator vessels and nerves lies medially

B) Ampulla of uterine tube on medial surface

C) Bifurcation of common iliac artery above

D) Ureter and internal iliac artery and vein behind

E) Posterior border of ovary lies free of mesovarium

Answer: a

59. True statement among following:

A) Uterus is maintain in anteverted position by transverse cervical ligament

B) Ureter lies above uterine vessels at level of isthmus

C) Patent processus vaginalis(canal of Nuck) leads to indirect inguinal hernia in female

D) Round ligament made up of smooth muscle fibres

E) Fallopian tube has inner longitudinal smooth muscle layer

Answer: c

60. Wrong statement among following is:

A) Vagina is lined by keratinized stratified squamous epithelium

B) Labia majora contain hair follicle, sebaceous and apocrine gland

C) Vestibule describe as area in between clitoris anteriorly, labia minora anteriorly, fourchette posteriorly and hymen superiorly

D) Greater vestibular gland of Bartholin`s open at 5 and 7 o`clock position posterolaterally at vaginal introitus

E) Nerve supply of vulva is iliohypogastric,ilioinguinal, and pudendal nerve

Answer: a

61. False statement about rectum is:

A) 15 cm long

B) Acute angulation is produce by   puborectalis

C) Has no taeniae or appendices epiploicae

D) Anterosuperiorly pouch of Douglas lies

E) Coloproctologist should be called if anorectal mucosal tear in vaginal delivery remain below puborectalis

Answer: e

62. False statement regarding anal canal is

A) It is 4 cm long and external anal sphincter is striated one (extension of voluntary levator ani muscle)

B) External anal sphincter is supplied by pudendal nerve

C) Internal anal sphincter is supplied by inferior hypogastric plexus and nervi erigentes

D) Below pectenline mucosa changes from columnar to squamous

E) Lymphatic drainage below intersphincteric groove is to rectum

Answer: e

63. False statement among following:

A) Urinary bladder is lined by transitional epithelium

B) Parasympathetic supply via splanchnics nerve is motor to detrusor and inhibitory to sphincter

C) Urethra cotain inner longitudinal smooth muscle layer which shorten during micturition and outer voluntary striated circular muscle which has a role in urinary incontinace

D) Breast is modified apocrine sweat gland

E) Growth of duct in breast is stimulated by progesteron

Answer: e

3.Biophysics

1. Soft markers of chromosomal abnormalities on ultrasound scan include:
   a) Echogenic bowel
   b) Mid renal pelvis dilation
   c) Choroid plexus cyst
   d) A,b,c
   e) Only a and c
      Answer: d

2. Ultrasound can cause:
   a) Cavitation
   b) Heating
   c) Micro-streaming
   d) No evidence of congenital abnormalities due to ultrasound yet
   e) All of above
      Answer: e

3. True statement about normal ECG:
   a) PR interval 0.2 to 0.4 sec
   b) Each QRS complex is preceded by p- wave
   c) The duration of QRS complex should be >0.12 sec
   d) The QT interval is 0.35 to 0.42 sec
   e) Paper speed is 1mm/sec
      Answer: b

4. Ultrasound determination of occiput before instrumental delivery increase rate of successful outcome:
   a) No
   b) Yes
   c) Cannot say
   d) Yes it is improved but definitive guidelines not yet established
   e) All of above
      Answer: d

5. Hysterosalpingography:
   a) Ultrasound is used
   b) Performed during menstrual phase of cycle
   c) Used to investigate infertility
   d) No need to do pregnancy test before hysteroslpingography
   e) It is contraindicated in patients with history of chlymydia and took treatment for same
   Answer: c

6. Parameters of fetal biophysical profile are:
   a) Non stress test
   b) Fetal breathing
   c) Fetal movement
   d) Amniotic fluid index and fetal tone
   e) All of above
   Answer: e

7. Which of following use ionizing form of radiation:
   a) Electrocautery
   b) Laser
   c) Magnetic resonance imagining
   d) Ultrasound
   e) X-ray
   Answer: e

8. X- ray exposure equivalent to
   a) 2-3 days
   b) 10 days
   c) 2 month
   d) 18 month
   e) 5 years
   Answer: a

9. Crown to rump length at which fetal heart sound is can be seen using ultrasound machine:
   a) >2mm
   b) >3mm
   c) >4mm

d) >5mm

e) >6mm

Answer: a

Table I. Components of the 30 minute Biophysical Profile Score	
Component	Definition
Fetal movements	≥ 3 body or limb movements
Fetal tone	One episode of active extension and flexion of the limbs; opening and closing of hand
Fetal breathing movements	≥1 episode of ≥30 seconds in 30 minutes - Hiccups are considered breathing activity.
Amniotic fluid volume	A single 2 cm x 2 cm pocket is considered adequate.
Non-stress test	2 accelerations > 15 beats per minute of at least 15 seconds duration.

Each of the 5 biophysical variables is currently scored as present (2 points) or absent (0 points). The total biophysical score obtained is either normal, equivocal, or abnormal (Table II). One advantage of the biophysical profile score as an antepartum test is the high percentage of normal test results. A normal biophysical profile score (8-10) occurs in 97.5% of cases (Table II)(Manning 1990b). There are fewer false positive tests with the biophysical profile score than with the non-stress test.

Table II. Distribution of Biophysical Profile Scores		
Score	Description	Percent
8 – 10	Normal	97.52
6	Equivocal	1.72
4	Abnormal	0.52
2	Abnormal	0.18
0	Abnormal	0.06

Definition of soft ultrasound markers

Soft markers are minor ultrasound abnormalities, considered variants of normal, which do not constitute a structural defect. They may be associated with chromosomal or none chromosomal abnormalities.

Soft markers include:

Those associated with increased risk of aneuploidy and in some cases none chromosomal problems: Nuchal translucency (NT), Nasal bone hypoplasia, Nuchal pad edema Echogenic bowel, Echogenic focus in the heart (golf ball sign), Choroid plexus cysts, Mild ventriculomegaly,

Those associated with an increased risk of non-chromosomal abnormalities when seen in isolation: Mild renal pyelectasis, Single umbilical artery, Enlarged cisterna

Those of undefined association: Clenched fists, Rocker bottom feet, Sandal gap, Strawberry shaped skull, Shortened long bones.

10.Defination of pregnancy failure is:
   a) Gestational sac >25 mm with no visible fetus

b) CRL> 7 mm with no cardiac activity

c) Fetal heart should be observed for 30 seconds

d) All of above

e) None of above

Answer: d

PREGNANCY FAILURE:

An experienced operator using high quality transvaginal equipment may diagnose pregnancy failure under either or both of the following circumstances:

1. When no live fetus is visible in a gestation sac and the mean sac diameter (MSD) cut off >25mm.

2. When there is a visible fetus with a CRL cut off >7mm but no fetal heart movements can be demonstrated. The area of the fetal heart should be observed for a prolonged period of at least thirty (30) seconds to ensure that there is no cardiac activity

Nuchal translucency :

It may be performed between the gestational ages of eleven (11) weeks and thirteen (13) weeks plus six (6) days (CRL 45-84mm). A measurement greater than 2.5-3 mm is usually considered to be abnormal but must be correlated with gestational age.

11. Nuchal translucency is abnormal when more than

a) 1mm

b) 2mm

c) 3mm

d) 5mm

e) 10 mm

Answer: c

X-rays during pregnancy carry a very small risk of exposing the unborn baby to radiation, which could cause cancer to develop during his or her childhood. The natural risk of childhood cancer is around 1 in 500. With low dose X-rays (below 10 mGy), the increased risk is very small (below 1 in 10,000). With higher dose X-rays (above 10 mGy), the increased risk is slightly higher, but remains low (mostly below 1 in 1,000).

4.Clinical managmet:

1. With regard to semen analysis:
   a) Men should abstain for 7 days before sample collection
   b) Collected sample should be deposited in laboratory within 48 hour
   c) Sperm should be collected in normal condom
   d) Semen analysis should be done to evaluate cause of infertility
   e) If it is abnormal should be repeated after 6 month
   Answer: d

2. HIV positive women wish to have normal vaginal delivery:
   a) Highly active antiretroviral treatment should be administered throughout labour
   b) Viral load should be less than 100 copies/ml
   c) Fetal blood sampling should be performed to assess fetal well being
   d) Membrane should be rupture as soon as possible
   e) Induction of labour is contraindicated
   Answer: a

3. About preconception conselling of women with pre-existing diabetes mellitus
   a) She should take 1000mcg of folic acid
   b) Statin should be started to lower lipid level
   c) HbA1c should be done every 6 weeks
   d) She should be discouraged to have pregnancy if hba1c is less than 8 %
   e) Metformin should be stop prior to conception

   Answer: c

4. Factor predisposing to post partum haemorrhage are:
   a) Multiple pregnancy
   b) Placenta previa
   c) Antepartum haemorrhage
   d) Polyhydroamnios
   e) All of above
   Answer: e

5. Primigravid 14 weeks of gestation come of routine antenatal check inform that her neighbor`s son have chickenpox and her varicella zoster virus IgG is positive . Correct statement regarding advice is:
   a) Chicken pox is not contagious disease
   b) She is immune to chicken pox so no action need to take
   c) She should not attend hospital as she may infect other patients
   d) She should undergo amniocentesis for diagnosis of fetal infection
   e) She should take varicella zoster immune globulin
   Answer: b

6. Primigravida 37 week presented with painless vaginal bleeding. Most probable diagnosis is:
   a) Abruption placentae
   b) Placenta previa
   c) Premature rupture of menmbrane
   d) Preterm labour
   e) Vasa previa
   Answer: b

7. 27 year old nulligravida presented with menorrhagia. First line of treatment should be:
   a) NSAIDS
   b) Oral contraceptive pills
   c) Dilation and curettage
   d) Levonorgestrol releasing intrauterine system
   e) Progesterone only pills

Answer: a

8. 30 year female presented with Dysmenorrhea with USG suggestive of 4 cm ovarian cyst. Rest of findings are normal. What is the appropriate management:
   a) Do MRI
   b) Laparoscopic cystectomy
   c) Reassure and discharge
   d) Serum ca-125
   e) Yearly USG follow-up
   Answer: c

9. 29 years old with history of pelvic inflammatory disease with known case of primary infertility , presently on clomiphene citrate for ovulation induction presented with pain in abdomen with bleeding per vaginum with pulse rate of 130 beats per minute and blood pressure 70/50mmhg. Urine pregnancy test positive most probable diagnosis is:
   a) Acute pelvic inflammatory disease
   b) Acute appendicitis
   c) Ruptured ectopic pregnancy
   d) Threatened miscarriage
   e) Urinary tract infection
   Answer: c

10. G2P1L1 35 week presented with blood pressure of 176/110mmhg and urine albumin positive, what is most appropriate line of management:
    a) Seizure prevention with magnesium sulfate
    b) Blood pressure control and continuation of pregnancy
    c) Seizure prevention, blood pressure control and immediate plan for delivery
    d) No need to do anything
    e) Diuretics before delivery
    Answer: c

11. RMI score include:
    a) Ultrasound score x menopausal status x CA 125 level

b) Ultrasound score x menopausal status

c) Only ultrasound score

d) Used to predict risk of ovarian cancer in women

e) A and d

Answer: e

12. A 45 years old premenopausal women presented with vaginal bleeding and HPE of endometrial biopsy suggestive of simple hyperplasia. Most appropriate management will be:

a) Hysterectomy

b) Hormonal replacement therapy with combined oral pills

c) Insertion of levonorgestrol- releasing intrauterine system

d) No treatment required

e) Ultrasound scan after 6 months

Answer: c

13. Mid wife unable to deliver baby after delivery of head. You are called for help. You made diagnosis of shoulder dystocia. What is most appropriate step:

a) Episiotomy

b) Fundal pressure

c) Traction on neck

d) McRobert's manoeuvre

e) Zavanelli manoeuvre

Answer: d

14. Primigravid 38 weeek presented with perceiving less fetal movement. What should be the first step to do:

a) Hear fetal heart sound using hand held dopler device

b) Do cardiotocography

c) Fetal blood sampling

d) Biophysical profile

e) Ultrasound

Answer: a

Features:	Baseline	Variability	Decelerations	Accelerations
Reassuring	110-160	>=5	None	Present
Non reassuring	100-109 162-180	< for >= 40 but less than 90 minute	Early deceleration variable deceleration single prolonged deceleration upto 3 minute	The absence of accelerations with an otherwise normal cardiotocograph is of uncertain singnificance
Abnormal	<100 >180 Sinusoidal pattern >=10minute	<5 for >= 90 minute	-Atypical variable decelerations -late decelerations -sinle prolonged decelerations greater than 3 minute	

Category	Definition
Normal	A cardiotocograph where all four fall into the reassuring category
Suspicious	A cardiotocograph whose features fall into one of the non-reassuring categories and the remainder of the features are reassuring
Pathological	A cardiotocograph whose features fall into two or more non reassuring categories or one or more abnormal categories

5. Embryology

1. Fertilization is the fusion of sperm and ovum to produce a zygote , it occurs in:
   a) Ampula
   b) Isthmus
   c) Fimbria
   d) Uterus
   e) Cornea
   Answer: a

2. Fertilization occur in ampula approximately _____ after ovulation:
   a) 1day
   b) 4days
   c) 1hour
   d) 12 hour
   e) 4hour
   Answer: d

3. Following fertilization ovum completed:
   a) First meiotic division and first polar body
   b) Second meiotic diviosion
   c) Second polar body
   d) Only a is correct
   e) Both b and c correct
   Answer: e
   Explanation:

Following fertilization the second meiotic division of the ovum is completed, leading to the production of a haploid ovum and the second polar body.

4. The first mitotic division of the zygote is achieved at
   a) 20 hour
   b) 30 hour
   c) 40 hour
   d) 50 hour
   e) 60 hour
   Answer: b

5. Gastrulation is process of :
   a) Development of three germ layer
   b) Fusion of sperm and ovum

c) Type of mitotic division
d) Formation of GIT
e) All of above
   Answer: a

6. Gastrulation occur in:
   a) 1 week
   b) 3 week
   c) 4 week
   d) 5 week
   e) 6 week
   Answer: b

7. First pair of somite appear by:
   a) Day 10 of intrauterine life
   b) Day 20 of intrauterine life
   c) Day 30 of intrauterine life
   d) Day 40 of intrauterine life
   e) Day 50 of intrauterine life
   Anwer: b

8. Neural plate appear by:
   a) Day 16
   b) Day 18
   c) Day 20
   d) Day 22
   e) Day 24
   Answer: b

9. Neural tube appear by:
   a) Day 16
   b) Day 18
   c) Day 20
   d) Day 22
   e) Day 24
   Answer: d

10.Cranial neuropore closes by:
   a) Day 16
   b) Day 18
   c) Day 20
   d) Day 22
   e) Day 24
   Answer: e

11.Caudal neuropore closes by:

a) Day 26
b) Day 18
c) Day 20
d) Day 22
e) Day 24
Answer:a

Gastrulation occurs in the third week of intra-uterine life. It give endoderm, mesoderm and ectoderm:
-the mesoderm is composed of the paraxial, intermediate, and lateral plate mesoderms.The paraxial mesoderms give rise to the somites rounded elevations of paraxial mesoderm that appear on either side of the neural tube under the surface ectoderm on the dorsal aspect of the embryo from the base of the skull to the tail region. The first pair appears on day 20 of intra-uterine life and they develop at a rate of three pairs per day to a maximum number of 42–44 pairs.
-neurulation is the formation of the nervous system and begins when the notochord induces the ectoderm germ layer to form the neural plate, which subsequently forms the neural tube .The neural plate may be seen by day 18 of intra- uterine life while the neural tube is seen by day 22 of intrauterine life.
-the neural tube later differentiates into the spinal cord and the brain. The openings of the neural tube at the cranial and caudal ends are called the cranial and caudal neuropores respectively.
-the cranial neuropore closes at day 24 while the caudal neuropore closes by day 26 of intra-uterine life. Failure of these closures leads to anencephaly and spinabifida respectively.

12. Urinary system develops from:
a) Ectoderm
b) Endoderm
c) Mesoderm
d) None of above
e) All of above
Answer: b

13. Nervous system develops from:
a) Ectoderm
b) Endoderm

    c) Mesoderm

    d) None of above

    e) All of above

       Answer: a

14. Connective tissue develops from:

    a) Ectoderm

    b) Endoderm

    c) Mesoderm

    d) None of above

    e) All of above

       Answer: c

Ectoderm
- epidermis
- nervous system

Mesoderm
- skeletal system and muscle
- connective tissues

Endoderm

- GIT
- Respiratory Tract
- Endocrine Glands
- Auditory System
- Urinary System

15. Septum secundum develops from:

    a) Atrial wall folding

    b) From septum primum

    c) Fossa ovalis

    d) Ventricular wall infolding

    e) None of above

       Answer: a

16. Truncus arteriosus give rise to:

    a) Pulmonary trunk

    b) Asending aorta

    c) Right ventricle

d) Both a and b

e) Both a and c

Answer: d

The atrial septum is formed in five stages and begins at about the fourth week of intra-uterine life.

1. Formation of the septum primum: this septum develops from the roof of the atrium anteriorly and grows towards the endocardial cushions. The septum is crescent-shaped and thus does not completely separate the two atrial chambers. This resultant gap is known as the ostium primum.

2. Closure of the ostium primum: as the septum primum develops, the ostium primum narrows and eventually closes.

3. Formation of the ostium secundum: this ostium forms on the septum primum as the ostium primum closes. It maintains the connection between the left and right atria.

4. Formation of the septum secundum: this septum forms to the right of the septum primum (figure 1.7 c). It originates from the posterior wall of the atria and grows over the septum primum leaving a small opening known as the foramen ovale (figure 1.7 d). The foramen ovale is continuous with the ostium secundum.

5. Regression of the septum primum: eventually the septum primum becomes the flap that covers the foramen ovale on its left side and is known as the valve of foramen ovale. After birth the foramen ovale becomes the fossa ovalis.

The ventricular septum is composed of two components:

1. A muscular part: this develops from the floor of theventricle and grows towards the endocardial cushions, but stops short of these and leaves a gap.

2. A membranous part: this is formed by the endocardial cushion and the aortopulmonary septum. It accommodates the atrioventricular conducting bundle.

● The cardiac outflowtract develops from the truncus

Arteriosus and bulbus cordis. The truncus arteriosus forms the ascending aorta and pulmonary trunk, whilst the bulbus cordis together with the primitive ventricle form the ventricles of the heart.

● The venous drainage of the heart consists of two sinuses, namely sinus venosum and sinus venarum.

● The arterial system comprises of a paired primitive aorta and the aortic arches. The primitive aorta is also known as the dorsal aorta and originates from the aortic sac. It is continuous with the umbilical artery posteriorly and the aortic arches anteriorly. They merge eventually to form the descending aorta.

17. Fetal lung maturation take place in:
    a) 1 stage
    b) 2 stage
    c) 3 stage
    d) 4 stage
    e) 5 stage
       Answer: e

18. Blood-air barrier in lung established in which phase:
    a) Glandular
    b) Canalicular
    c) Saccular
    d) Alveolar
    e) After birth
       Answer: c

19. Primiary alveoli develops in:
    a) Glandular
    b) Canalicular
    c) Saccular
    d) Alveolar
    e) After birth
       Answer: b

20. Between 6 to 16 week there is:
    a) Glandular
    b) Canalicular
    c) Saccular
    d) Alveolar
    e) After birth
       Answer: a

21. Most of component of blood develops in:
    a) Glandular
    b) Canalicular
    c) Saccular
    d) Alveolar
    e) After birth
       Answer: a

22. Surfactant secreted by:

a) Type i pneumocytes after birth
b) Type ii pneumocytes after birth
c) Type i pneumocytes at 24 week
d) Type ii pneumocytes at 24 week
e) Squamous epithelial cells
   Answer: d

Fetal lung maturation has four stages known as the glandular,canalicular, saccular, and alveolar periods. The glandular period occurs between 6 to 16 weeks of intra-uterine life. During this period most of the lung components are formed, except for the alveoli. Hence, gaseous exchange is not possible at the end of this period. The alveoli tend to develop in the canalicular period that occurs between 16 to 24 weeks of intra-uterine life. The saccular period is between 24 weeks of intra-uterine life to birth. It is during this period that the blood-air barrier is established and specialized cells of the respiratory epithelium appear. The blood-air barrier is also known as the alveolar-capillary

Barrier. There are two types of lung cells:
• type 1 pneumocytes that line the alveoli
• type 2 pneumocytes that appear at 24 weeks of intrauterine life and are responsible for surfactant production.

23. Diaphragm is made up of:
   a) Septum transversum
   b) The body wall
   c) Mesentery of the oesophagus
   d) Pleuroperitoneal membrane
   e) All of above.
Answer: e

24. Structure passing through oesophageal hiatus is:
   a) Oesophagus and vagal trunk
   b) Inferior vena cava
   c) Right phrenic nerve
   d) Aorta
   e) Superior epigastric vein
      Answer: a

25. Structure passing through diaphragm at level T12 is:

a) Oesophagus and vagal trunk
b) Inferior vena cava
c) Right phrenic nerve
d) Aorta
e) Superior epigastric vein

Answer: d

26. Structure passing through caval opening is:
a) Oesophagus and vagal trunk
b) Right phrenic nerve
c) Right phrenic nerve
d) Aorta
e) Superior epigastric vein

Answer: b

The diaphragm is composed of five components :
• Septum transversum
• The body wall
• Mesentery of the oesophagus
• Pleuroperitoneal membrane
• Third, fourth, and fifth cervical somites.

Structures that pass through the diaphragm and their transmitting channels:
•Caval opening (T8) — inferior vena cava and right phrenic nerve
• Oesophageal hiatus (T10) — oesophagus and vagal trunk
•Aortic hiatus (T12) — aorta, azygous vein, and thoracic duct
• Foramen of morgagni (Larrey's triangle) — superior epigastric vessels
• Apertures of right crus — right splanchnic nerve
• Apertures of left crus — left splanchnic nerve and hemiazygous vein.

27. Structure develops in foregut are:
a) Oesophagus
b) Stomach
c) Duodenum

d) Pancrease

e) All of above

Answer: e

28. Foregut is supplied by:

a) Coeliac trunk

b) Superior mesenteric artery

c) Inferior mesenteric artery

d) Inferior rectal artery

e) Perineal artery

Answer: a

29. Midgut is supplied by:

a) Coeliac trunk

b) Superior mesenteric artery

c) Inferior mesenteric artery

d) Inferior rectal artery

e) Perineal artery

Answer: b

30. Hindgut is supplied by:

a) Coeliac trunk

b) Superior mesenteric artery

c) Inferior mesenteric artery

d) Inferior rectal artery

e) Perineal artery

Answer: c

The foregut begins at the mouth and ends at the entrance of the bile duct into the duodenum. It includes the oesophagus, stomach, duodenum, pancreas, and liver.

The midgut begins from the opening of the bile duct and ends about two-thirds of the way along the transverse colon. Its vascular supply arises from the superior mesenteric artery. The hindgut runs from the distal third of the transverse colon to the upper half of the anal canal. It derives its arterial supply from the inferior mesenteric artery. Initially the hindgut opens into the primitive cloaca, the precursor to the bladder (urogenital sinus), and the rectum (hindgut).

31.Dorsal mesentry is absent over:
a) Oesophagus
b) Stomach
c) Small bowel
d) Transverse colon
e) Duodenum
Answer: e

The dorsal mesentery extends from the lower esophagus to the cloaca but is lost over the duodenum, ascending colon, and descending colon.The ventral mesentery is smaller than the dorsal mesentery. It arises from the septum transversum and Covers the stomach, terminal oesophagus, and initial Portion of duodenum. The liver develops within the Ventral mesentery while the spleen arises from the Dorsal mesogastrium. The pancreas develops from endodermal lining of the duodenum starting as Two pancreatic buds, the dorsal and ventral buds, which begin to arise from week 4 of intra-uterine life. The dorsal bud lies within the dorsal mesentery and is larger of the two buds, while the ventral bud lies within the ventral mesentery.

32.Liver start producing red blood cells around:
a) 8 week of intrauterine life
b) 10 week of intrauterine life
c) 12 week of intrauterine life
d) 14 week of intrauterine life
e) 16 week of intrauterine life
Answer: b

The hepatic diverticulum arises above the pancreatic Duct from the ventral wall of the duodenum. By week 10 of intra-uterine life the liver starts producing red Blood cells. Prior to this the red blood cells contain a Nucleus and are produced by the mesoblast.

33.Herniation of gut is reduce by:
a) 8 week of intrauterine life
b) 10 week of intrauterine life
c) 12 week of intrauterine life
d) 14 week of intrauterine life
e) 16 week of intrauterine life

Answer: b

Through fetal development the midgut rapidly elongates and outgrows the small volume of the peritoneal cavity. This leads to the herniation of the midgut via the umbilical cord at around 6 weeks of intra-uterine life . As the midgut herniates out of the peritoneal cavity it rotates 90 ° anticlockwise along its long axis. This process is known as physiological herniation. The herniation is reduced at 10 weeks of intra-uterine life when the volume of the peritoneal cavity is bigger than the length of the midgut. As the herniated midgut reduces into the peritoneal cavity it rotates a further 180 ° anticlockwise on its mesentery. These rotational movements explain the final positions
Of intra-abdominal organs in adult life.

34. Median umbilical ligament is remnant of :
    a) Allantois
    b) Septum primum
    c) Right umbilical artery
    d) Left umbilical artery
    e) Uterine artery
       Answer: a
35. Cloacal membrane breaks at:
    a) 5 week
    b) 7 week
    c) 9 week
    d) 11 week
    e) 13 week
       Answer: b

The allantois is initially continuous with the bladder, but as the bladder enlarges with further development and division of the urogenital sinus and the hindgut by the urorectal septum, the allantois constricts and becomes a thick, fibrous cord called the urachus, represented in the adult as the median umbilical ligament.This remnant structure lies in the space of retzius, between the transversalis fascia anteriorly and the peritoneum posteriorly.The blood vessels of the allantois become the umbilical arteries and vein. The cloacal membrane breaks down at week 7 of intra-uterine life.

36. Lumen of anal canal recanalize at
   a) 5 week
   b) 7 week
   c) 9 week
   d) 11 week
   e) 13 week
      Answer: c

37. Upper two third of anal canal is derived from endoderm. It is lined by:
   a) Stratified squamous epithelium
   b) Non stratified squamous epithelium
   c) Columnar epithelium
   d) Cuboidal epithelium
   e) Transitional epithelium
      Answer: c

38. Lower third of anal canal is derived from endoderm. It is lined by:
   a) Stratified squamous epithelium
   b) Non stratified squamous epithelium
   c) Columnar epithelium
   d) Cuboidal epithelium
   e) Transitional epithelium
      Answer: a

The anal canal is derived from two embryological tissues demarcated by the pectinate line. The upper part of the anal canal is derived from endoderm while the lower part is derived from ectoderm. Thus, the upper two-thirds are lined with columnar epithelium and derive their blood supply from the superior rectal artery (which is a branch of the inferior mesenteric artery). The lower third, however, is lined with stratified squamous epithelium and derives its blood supply from the inferior rectal artery (which is a branch of the Internal pudendal artery). The lumen of the anal canal is initially occluded at 7 weeks of intra-uterine life and recanalized at 9 weeks.

39. True about pronephron and mesonephron is:

a) Appear at 22 weeks of intrauterine life
b) Transient and replaced by mesonephron
c) Cavity in mesonephron form Bowmen`s capsule
d) Join laterally to form mesonephric duct and drain into urogenital sinus and form triagone
e) All of above
Answer: e

The development of a kidney proceeds through three
Main phases:
• pronephros: appears by day 22 of intra-uterine life
• mesonephros
• metanephros: appears by fifth week of intra-uterine life.
■ pronephros is a rudimentary organ that appears at the end of the third week of intra-uterine life. It is transient and is replaced by the mesonephros.The mesonephros develops in the lower thoracic and lumbar region. The cavities that appear in the Mesonephros become the Bowman's capsule and join laterally to form the mesonephric duct .these ducts drain into the urogenital sinus and form the bladder trigone.

40. In male mesonephric duct form:
a) Ductus deferens
b) Gartner`s duct
c) Prostate
d) Bladder
e) Bartholin`s gland
Answer: a

The male the mesonephric ducts also give rise to the ductus deferens and the efferent ductules of the testes. In the female they produce the Gardner's ducts.

41. False statement among following is:
a) Metanephron form definitive kidney
b) Ureteric bud begins to develop from 5 weeks of intrauterine life
c) Metanehric blastima form nephron
d) Nephron develops till term
e) Nephron fuction as early as 10 weeks of intrauterine life

Answer: d

42. Metanphric duct form:
    a) Renal pelvis
    b) Ureter
    c) Calyces
    d) Collecting duct
    e) All of above
    Answer: e

The metanephros eventually becomes the definitive adult kidney. It consists of the ureteric bud and the metanephric blastema. The ureteric bud is an outgrowth of the mesonephric duct and begins to develop from week 5 of intra-uterine life. It eventually grows into the metanephric duct, which then forms the:

1. Definitive ureter
2. Renal pelvis
3. Calyces
4. Collecting ducts.

The metanephric blastema is the condensation ofNephrogenic cord tissue around the ureteric bud and forms the nephrons. Formation of the nephrons continues until 32 weeks of intra-uterine life. The nephrons are functional from as early as 10 weeks of Intra-uterine life.

43. Urogenital sinus does not form:
    a) Bladder
    b) Prostate
    c) Bartholin`s gland
    d) Collecting duct
    e) Skene`s gland
    Answer: d

The bladder arises from the urogenital sinus after the division of the cloaca. The urogenital sinus also forms the Bartholin's glands and Skene's glands, which are analogous to the male prostate. It has three portions:

1. Vesico-ureteric: forms the bladder
2. Pelvic: forms the prostate
3. Phallic.

The urogenital sinus is initially continuous with the allantois. **After birth the allantois degenerates to become the urachus, forming the median umbilical ligament.**

44. Development of female reproductive system requires:
    a) Presence of testosterone
    b) Presence of estrogen
    c) Absence of testosterone and presence of anti mullerian hormone
    d) Presence of testosterone and presence of anti mullerian hormone
    e) Absence of ant-mullerian hormone and absence of testosterone

    Answer: e

The development of the female internal genitalia occurs in the absence of testosterone and anti-mullerian hormone. At first, the mesonephric and paramesonephric ducts arises.

The mesonephric ducts (commonly known as the wolffian ducts) persist in the male and regress in the female due to the effect of circulating testosterone, which begins in the **male fetus by 8 weeks of intra-uterine life.** They connect to the urogenital sinus and lose their urinary function once the metanephros is formed. The mesonephric

Duct is responsible for the formation of the:

- Ductus deferens
- Epididymis
- Seminal vesicles
- Prostatic utricle
- Trigone of the bladder.

45. Paramesonephric duct does not form:
    a) Fallopian tube
    b) Broad ligament
    c) Lower vagina
    d) Uterus
    e) Cervix

    Answer: c

• The paramesonephric ducts are also known as the mullerian ducts. Unlike the mesonephric ducts, they persist in the female and regress in the male. Regression of these ducts is due to the secretion of anti-mullerian hormone in the male fetus. The ducts lie lateral to the mesonephric ducts and form the:

■ fallopian tubes
■ broad ligament
■ uterovaginal canal.

● the uterovaginal canal gives rise to the uterus, cervix, and upper half of the vagina. It eventually fuses with the sinovaginal bulb, which is the swelling on the urogenital sinus that forms the lower half of the vagina and the vaginal plate.

46. External genitalia is indifferentiated upto:
    a) 7 week
    b) 8 week
    c) 9 week
    d) 10 week
    e) 11 week
       Answer: c

47. Wrong pair from following:
    a) Genital tubercle: clitoris
    b) Genital fold: labia minora
    c) Genital swelling: labia majora
    d) Sex cord development: 4 week
    e) Ova: develops from primordial germ cells which migrate from yolk sac
       Answer: d

The external genitalia are undiffirentiated until **9 weeks of** intra-uterine life. The **default development is towards the female phenotype in the absence of dihydrotestosterone (DHT). At about 5 weeks of intra-uterine life a cloacal fold forms on either side of the cloacal membrane.** This fold forms the labia minora in females and the penile urethra in males. The fusion of the cloacal folds anteriorly gives rise to the genital tubercle. The genital tubercle elongates to form the clitoris in the female fetus and gives rise to the penis in the male fetus. Lateral to the cloacal folds are the genital swellings that form the labia majora or scrotum in the female or male fetus respectively.

● the development of the gonads starts in the form of a common primordium in the genital ridges adjacent to the developing kidney at around **4 weeks** of intra-uterine life. At around **6**

weeks of intra-uterine life, sex cords develop within the forming gonads. Later in intrauterine life they differentiate into the male (testis) and female (ovary) sex organs. **The differentiation into the testes is determined by the presence of the SRY gene on the Y chromosome.**

• The ovary is formed by the gonadal ridge and mesonephros. It consists of a medulla and a surface germinal epithelium and contains the ova. The ova originate from the primordial germ cells that migrate from the endoderm of the yolk sac via the hindgut to the genital ridge.

48. Wrong statement among following is:
    a) Sertoli cell secrets mullerian hormone
    b) Leydig cell produce testosteron
    c) Testosterone and antimullerian hormone secreted as early as 8 week of intrauterine life
    d) Testes are guided into scrotum by gubernaculum
    e) Second phase of testes descent is independent of hormone
    Answer: e

• The testes comprise of two primary cells: sertoli and Leydig cells. The sertoli cells secrete the anti-mullerian Hormone while the leydig cells produce testosterone. These hormonal secretions begin as early as 8 weeks of intra-uterine life.

• The testes are guided in their descent towards the labioscrotal swelling by the gubernaculum during fetal maturation. This descent comprises of two phases. The first phase is an independent phase that occurs until the testes reach the deep inguinal ring at about 7 months of intrauterine life. The second phase is hormone dependent and occurs from 7 to 9 months of intra-uterine life. **The gubernaculum in female fetuses becomes the ovarian and round ligaments**.

49. Wrong statement about placental development:
    a) Trophoblast form placenta and differentiated into syncytiotrophoblast and cytotrophoblast
    b) The chorionic villi increase the surface area available for gaseous and substrate exchange with the maternal blood.
    c) Primary villi contain trophoblast and mesoderm

d) Secondary villi contain trophoblast and mesoderm
e) Tertiary villi contain trophoblast , mesoderm and blood vessels

Answer: c

The choriodecidual interface is a functional fetomaternal organ and has two parts:

● Chorion frondosum (the fetal part)
● Decidua basalis (the maternal part).

■The placenta begins its development from implantation and is derived from the trophoblast of the blastocyst. **Trophoblastic differentiation gives rise to the cytotrophoblast and syntiotrophoblast.**

■ The functional component of the placenta is the chorionic villi. **The chorionic villi increase the surface area available for gaseous and substrate exchange with the maternal blood**. It is the chorionic villi that are responsible for uterine decidual invasion. With time, the primary chorionic villi develop into the secondary and tertiary chorionic villi with the inclusion of mesoderm and blood vessels.

1. Primary: contains only trophoblast
2. Secondary: contains trophoblast and mesoderm
3. Tertiary: contains trophoblast, mesoderm, and
Blood vessels

50. Wrong statement regarding fibrinoid deposition in placenta is:
a) Fibrinoid deposition occur in subchorial Langhan`s layer
b) Fibrinoid deposition occur in subchorial Rohr`s layer
c) Nitabutch`s layer
d) Through Rohr`s layer placenta separate after birth
e) Fetal membrane include amniotic membrane, yolk sac , chorion, allantois

Answer: d

■ fibrinoid deposition occurs in the placenta from as early as 4 months of gestation. Accumulation of the fibrin occurs in three regions of the placenta:

1. Subchorial langhan's layer within the chorion plate
2. Rohr's layer beneath the stem villi within the basal plate
3. Nitabutch's layer in the decidua basalis within the basal plate **(this is the layer from which the placenta detaches at birth).**

■ 'fetal membranes' is the term applied to structures derived from the blastocyte that do not contribute to the embryo. They are made up of the amnion,Chorion, yolk sac, and allantois. The amnion has no blood vessels, lymphatics, or nerves and consists of

Five layers:

1. Cuboidal epithelium
2. Basement membrane
3. Compact layer
4. Fibroblast layer
5. Spongy layer (remnant of extra-embryonic Coelom).

■ the chorion is composed of four layers:

1. Cellular layer
2. Reticular layer
3. Basement membrane
4. Trophoblast.

6.Endocrinology:

1. Which of following is wrong statement abut hormones:
   a) Protein hormones present in bound form in circulation
   b) Protein hormones half life is in minute
   c) Steroid hormone present in boud form in circulation
   d) Steroid hormone receptors are intracellular
   e) Protein hormone receptors are present on outer surface of cell membrane

Answer: a

There are three main chemical classes of hormones.

1. Protein and peptide hormones

Half lives in the circulation are in the order of minutes and they generally circulate unbound and in free form *except for IGF-1* , which is strongly bound to the binding protein IGFBP-1 and so has a long half life. Protein and peptide hormones, catecholamines, and Melatonin (biogenic amine hormones) are hydrophilic (water soluble) and do not cross the lipid bilayer of cell Membranes.

Their receptors are resident on the outer surface of the Cell membrane and their intracellular actions are exerted by secondary messengers such as CAMP.

They are stored within intracellular vesicles as prohormones.

2. Steroid hormones

● These are highly conserved and are derived from cholesterol.

● They are secreted from the adrenal cortex, ovaries, testes, and the kidneys (the active form of vitamin d).

● Their plasma transport involves binding to specific transport proteins and albumin, because unlike peptide hormones they cannot dissolve in the aqueous medium of plasma. As a result their half lives are long and in the order of hours to days. The length of the half life is proportional to the affinity of the hormone for the binding protein. The very small unbound fraction is the biologically active form.

● Steroid and thyroid hormones are hydrophobic and readily cross the lipid bilayer of cell membranes.

• Their receptors are mainly intracellular and their biologic actions are exerted by generating brand new intracellular proteins, which in part explains why they take longer to act.

• Unlike protein and peptide hormones, steroid hormones are not stored in intracellular vesicles but are synthesized and released as required.

3. Hormones derived from an amino acid

• The catecholamines secreted by the adrenal medulla are tyrosine derivatives whilst melatonin secreted by the pineal is derived from tryptophan.

• Catecholamines circulate in free form and their half lives are in the order of seconds.

Thyroid hormones are derived from two bound tyrosine molecules that are Iodinated but like steroids they are mainly bound in the Circulation and have long half lives.

2. Which of the following hormone secreted from acidophilic cells of pituitary gland:
   a) FSH
   b) LH
   c) TSH
   d) GH
   e) ACTH

Answer: d

3. Which of following hormone secreted from posterior pituitary:
   a) ACTH
   b) TSH
   c) Oxytocin
   d) LH
   e) FSH

Answer: c

Cells of the adenohypophysis are chromophils (acidophils and basophils, according to the histological dyes they take up) and chromophobes, which are generally considered to be non-secretory.

The posterior lobe of the pituitary gland originates from neural tissue and consists of the nerve terminals of neurosecretory cells whose cell bodies lie in the supraoptic and paraventricular nuclei of the hypothalamus. Here they synthesize and package oxytocin and vasopressin (VP), otherwise known as antidiuretic hormone (ADH). The secretor vesicles containing the hormones are transported down the axons that pass through the neural stalk, and are stored in the nerve terminals in the posterior pituitary gland.

Anterior pituitary secrets:

- Growth hormone (GH) from somatotrophs (acidophils) — 50 %
- Prolactin (PRL) from lactotrophs (acidophils) — 10–15 % (increasing in pregnancy)
- Thyroid-stimulating hormone (TSH) from thyrotrophs (basophils) — 3–5 %
- Adenocorticotrophic hormone (ACTH) from corticotrophs(basophils — 15–20 %)
- Gonadotrophins, Luteinizing hormone (LH), and Folliclestimulating hormone (FSH) from gonadotrophs (basophils) — 10 % .

4. Wrong statement about growth hormone is:
   a) Made up of 192 amino acid
   b) Pulse amplitude increases at onset of sleep
   c) Inhibited by insulin like growth factor
   d) Inhibited by hypoglycemia
   e) IGF-1 is good index of 24hour GH secretion.

Answer: d

Growth hormone

192 amino acids, that is structurally similar to prolactin. Its synthesis and secretion are stimulated by growth hormone-releasing hormone (GHRH) and inhibited by somatostatin, both of which are released by neurosecretory cells in the hypothalamus. TheirIntegrated actions result in the secretion of

discrete pulses of GH throughout the day (approximately six pulses) with an increased pulse amplitude related to the onset of sleep.

GH pulse frequency and secretion is high during puberty and declines in senescence.

Stimulation – GHRH, hypoglycaemia, decreased free fatty acids, starvation, sleep exercise, stress, puberty Oestrogens and androgens, alpha adrenergic agonists, and dopamine agonists.

Inhibition – somatostatin, hyperglycaemia, increased free fatty acids, insulin-like growth factors (IGFS), growth hormone (short loop feedback), progesterone, glucocorticoids, beta adrenergic agonists, and dopamine (DA) antagonists .

Actions of GH

● GH has short-term (acute stress response) actions, which are direct, and long-term indirect (anabolic) actions.

● GH raises plasma glucose by directly stimulating gluconeogenesis in the liver and reducing the uptake of glucose in peripheral tissues. It mobilizes fat and increases circulating free fatty acids by stimulating the action of *hormone sensitive lipase,* a major mobilizer of fat from adipose tissues.

● long-term anabolic GH actions are mediated through the stimulation of the synthesis and secretion of IGF and IGF-binding proteins (IGFBPS) from the liver. GH stimulates the uptake of amino acids for protein synthesis and increases lean body mass. IGFS stimulate somatic cell growth with an increase in the size and function of organs and tissues. IGF have a (long-loop) negative feedback effect on GH secretion.

● IGF-1 is a relatively good index of plasma GH 24-hour secretion because GH itself is released in a pulsatile fashion and IGF-1 has a long half life.

    5. Prolactin secretion inhibited by:
      a) Dopamine
      b) TRH
      c) Suckling
      d) Pregnancy
      e) Dopamine antagonist

Answer: a

Prolactin
- Unlike all other anterior pituitary hormones, the predominant hypothalamic control of prolactin secretion is inhibitory through dopamine (DA) secreted by neurosecretory cells.
- Secretion is stimulated by TRH, pregnancy, lactation (suckling), oestrogens, opioids, stress, and dopamine antagonists. Prolactin is secreted in a pulsatile fashion and the amplitude of pulses increases with the onset of sleep.
- The major function of prolactin is the stimulation of breast development and milk production in females, although males have the same circulating concentrations of prolactin.

6. Wrong statement about thyroid hormone is:
   a) 70% bound to thyroid binding globulin
   b) Half life of t3 1 week
   c) 15% bound to albumin
   d) Half life of t4 1 week
   e) 15% bound to prealbumin

Answer: b

7. Mineralocorticoid produce from:
   a) Zona glomerulosa
   b) Zona fasciculata
   c) Zona reticularis
   d) Adrenal medulla
   e) Ovary

Answer: a

8. Glucocorticoid produce from:
   a) Zona glomerulosa
   b) Zona fasciculata
   c) Zona reticularis
   d) Adrenal medulla
   e) Ovary

Answer: b

9. Androgen produce from:
   a) Zona glomerulosa
   b) Zona fasciculata

    c) Zona reticularis

    d) Adrenal medulla

    e) Ovary

Answer: c

10. Adrenalin produce from:

    a) Zona glomerulosa

    b) Zona fasciculata

    c) Zona reticularis

    d) Adrenal medulla

    e) Ovary

Answer: d

11. Aldosterone produce from:

    a) Zona glomerulosa

    b) Zona fasciculata

    c) Zona reticularis

    d) Adrenal medulla

    e) Ovary

Answer: a

12. Aldosterone act on:

    a) PCT

    b) DCT

    c) DCT and collecting duct

    d) Vasa recti

    e) Collecting duct

Answer: c

13. Angiotensinogen is produce from:

    a) Zona glomerulosa

    b) Zona fasciculata

    c) Zona reticularis

    d) Adrenal medulla

    e) Liver

Answer: e

14. Renin secreted from:

a) Zona glomerulosa
b) Zona fasciculata
c) Zona reticularis
d) Juxtaglomerular appratus
e) Ovary

Answer: d

15. Angiotensinogen to angiotensin 1 is converted by:
a) ACE
b) Renin
c) Aldosteron
d) Adrenalin
e) Oestrogen

Answer: b

16. Fetal adrenal cortex develops from:
a) Endoderm
b) Ectoderm
c) Mesoderm
d) Neural crest cells
e) Yolk sac

Answer: c

The fetal adrenal cortex develops from the coelomic mesoderm whilst the adrenal medulla is formed from an adjacent sympathetic ganglion that is derived from neural crest cells.

17. Most common enzyme responsible for female pseudohermaphrodism is:
a) 21-hydroxylase
b) 3 beta hydroxylase
c) 11 hydroxylase
d) 17,20 lyase
e) P450

Answer: a

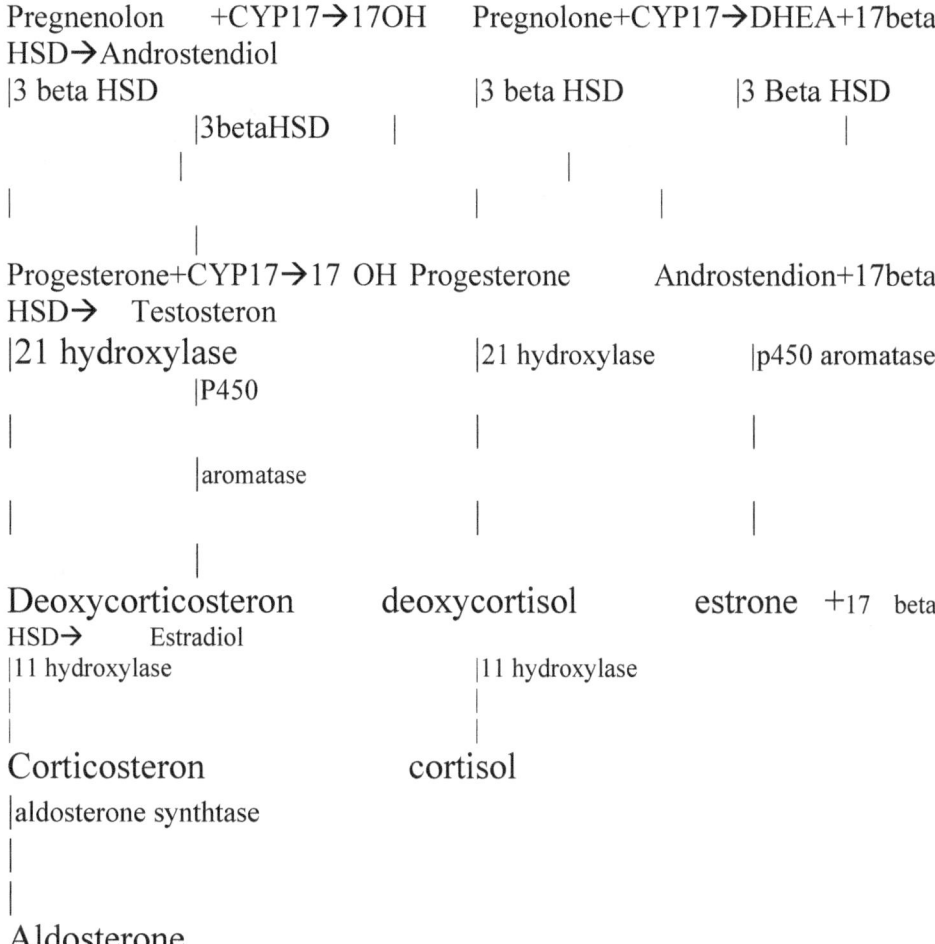

Pregnenolon   +CYP17→17OH   Pregnolone+CYP17→DHEA+17beta
HSD→Androstendiol
|3 beta HSD |3 beta HSD |3 Beta HSD
            |3betaHSD |
            | |
| | |
            |
Progesterone+CYP17→17 OH Progesterone   Androstendion+17beta
HSD→   Testosteron
|21 hydroxylase |21 hydroxylase |p450 aromatase
            |P450
| | |
            |aromatase
| | |
            |
Deoxycorticosteron   deoxycortisol   estrone +17 beta
HSD→   Estradiol
|11 hydroxylase |11 hydroxylase
| |
| |
Corticosteron   cortisol
|aldosterone synthtase
|
|
Aldosterone

18. 40 year obese female with hypertension presented with depression and purple stria on abdomen, most likely diagnosis is:
    a) Hyperthyroidism
    b) ACTH deficiency
    c) Cushing`s syndrome
    d) Hypothyroidism
    e) 21 hydroxylase deficiency

Answer: c

• Excess cortisol secretion (cushing's syndrome/disease) caused by an endogenous source (e.g. ACTH-secreting Pituitary adenoma or adrenal tumour) or by exogenous steroidal anti-infl ammatory drugs results in proximal myopathy, bruising, scarring, and purple striae round the abdomen, loss of bone mass, hypertension, and Depression.

• Primary adrenocortical deficiency — Addison's disease — causes low systolic blood pressure, weight loss due to reduced appetite, and skin pigmentation due to excess ACTH (reduction of negative feedback), which interacts with melanocortin receptors in the skin

19. Regarding vitamin D false statement is:
  a) Increase cacium level
  b) 7 dehydrocholesterol convert into cholecalciferol by ultraviolet light in skin
  c) 25 hydroxylation occur in liver
  d) 1,25 hydroxylation occur in kidney
  e) Parathhormone increase calcium absorption from gut

Answer: e

20. Process of maturation of sperm from spematogonia occur in
  a) 5-6 week
  b) 7-8 week
  c) 8-9 week
  d) 9-10 week
  e) 10-11 week

Answer: d

21. Supporting cells for spermatogenesis is:
  a) Leydig`s cell
  b) Sertoli cell
  c) Seminiferous tubule epithelial cells
  d) Follicular cells
  e) Prostatic cells

Answer: b

Spermatogenesis is 'nurtured' by the sertoli cells, which organize waves of spermatogenesis.

22. Sertoli cell functions are:

a) Secret AMH
b) Secret inhbin
c) Have aromatase activity
d) Secret androgen binding protein
e) All of above

Answer: e

Sertoli cells synthesize and secrete androgen-binding protein into the seminiferous tubules, which binds up testosterone to about 50-fold the concentration found in plasma. The target cell of FSH in the adult male is the sertoli cell, which is absolutely essential for sperm development. Sertoli cells possess aromatase activity and therefore convert androgens to oestrogens, and also transport sperm into the lumen of the seminiferous tubules and produce inhibin, which exerts a negative feedback effect on FSH secretion at the level of the pituitary gland.

23. 95% of testosterone secreted from:
    a) Adrenal gland
    b) Ovary
    c) Adipose tissue
    d) Testes
    e) Pituitary

Answer: d

24. False statement among following is:
    a) LH act on leydig cell and produce testosteron
    b) FSH act on sertoli cell
    c) 2% testosterone is free in circulation
    d) 60% of testosterone bound to albumin
    e) Action of testosterone is exerted by dihydrotestosteron

Answer: d

Testosterone is synthesized and secreted by the leydig cells in response to LH. Up to 95 % of circulating testosterone is derived from the testis, and the rest from peripheral conversion of adrenal androgens.

• Only 2 % of circulating testosterone is in the free form; the rest is either bound to albumin (~40 %) or SHBG (~60%).

• Under normal conditions, testosterone exerts negative feedback effects on LH secretion (not on FSH) and testosterone is important in the development and maintenance of the reproductive tract.

• The actions of testosterone on the penis, scrotum, and prostate and other peripheral tissues are dependent on its conversion to the more active form dihydrotestosterone (DHT) by the enzyme 5 alpha-reductase in target cells.

25. Maximum number of follicle is present at _____ :
   a) 10 week of gestation
   b) 20 week of gestation
   c) At menopause
   d) At birth
   e) At menarch

Answer: b

The maximum number of primordial follicles in the ovary is achieved at 20 weeks' gestation when it is approximately 7 million, and decreases progressively from this point such that at birth each ovary contains about 2 million primordial follicles and 300 000 by menarche. Primordial follicles consist of a single oocyte halfway through its first meiotic division and surrounded by a flattened layer of granulosa cells.

26. False statement about follicular phase of menstrual cycle is:
   a) Oestrogen increases as cycle progress
   b) When oestrogen reaches at >750pmol/l negative feedback converts into positive feedback
   c) Positive feedback cause FSH peak
   d) Ovulation occur 12 hour after LH surge
   e) FSH stimulates growth of preantral and antral follicle

Answer: c

Follicular phase

- This begins with the first day of menstruation and is associated with a rise in FSH secretion that stimulates the growth and differentiation of cohorts of preantral and antral follicles. As a result oestrogen synthesis and secretion rises, reaching a peak at mid-cycle, whilst LH and FSH secretions decline (negative feedback)
- when oestrogen levels reach a peak concentration (> 750 pmol/l) sustained for 24–48 h, oestrogen no longer provides negative feedback but switches to a positive feedback effect on GNRH/gonadotrophin secretion, resulting in a pre-ovulatory surge of LH and a smaller surge of FSH. This induces completion of the first meiotic division of the oocyte (to give a mature oocyte and polar body) and initiation of the second meiotic division. Ovulation occurs 9–12 hours after the LH surge. Only the LH surge is required for ovulation.

27. In pregnancy corpus luteum is maintain by:

    a) LH

    b) FSH

    c) hCG

    d) Oestrogen

    e) Progesteron

Answer: c

Luteal phase

- The granulosa and thecal cells of the empty follicle rapidly proliferate and form the corpus luteum. The corpus luteum synthesizes progesterone and to a lesser extent oestradiol. During the luteal phase, progesterone provides the major feedback to LH secretion.
- Small amounts of gonadotrophins, particularly LH, are required to maintain the secretory activity of the corpusluteum but, in the absence of conception, the corpus luteum undergoes luteolysis (a process not well defined but believed to be apoptotic) about 14 days after ovulation.
- The loss of negative feedback from oestradiol and progesterone induces the intercycle rise in FSH secretion and another cycle begins.

• If conception occurs the corpus luteum does not undergo luteolysis but is maintained by human chorionic gonadotrophin (HCG) secreted by the developing placenta.

28. Androgen and progesterone produced by theca cells under action of LH. Androgen converted into estrogen by:
    a) Theca cell under action of LH
    b) Theca cell under action of FSH
    c) Granulosa cells under action of LH
    d) Granulosa cells under action of FSH
    e) None of above

Answer: d

Progesterone and androgen production in thecal cells is stimulated by LH.
• The androgens diffuse across the basement membrane into the granulosa cell layer where, under the influence of FSH, the androgens are converted to oestrogens under the action of aromatase.
• Just prior to ovulation, granulosa cells develop LH receptors and can respond to the pre-ovulatory surge of LH. Steroid secretions of the corpus luteum are mainly stimulated by LH.

29. Estradiol and progesterone are not transported in circulation by:
    a) Albumin
    b) Sex hormone binding gloulin
    c) Cortisol binding globulin
    d) Pre-albumin
    e) 2% free form

Answer: d

• Oestradiol and progesterone are transported in the circulation bound to sex hormone-binding globulin (SHBG) and albumin, with progesterone having a low affinity for SHBG but a higher affinity for cortisol-binding globulin. About 2 % of these hormones exist in free form in the circulation.

30. False statement about hormonal changes during puberty is:

a) Rise in adrenal androgen at 6 to 8 years
b) Increase in amplitude and frequency GNRH pulse.
c) Adipose tissue secret leptin
d) Kisspeptin release from hypothalamic neurons
e) All of above

Answer: e

Hormonal changes in puberty

The endocrinology of puberty consists of two phases:

1. Adrenarche: the rise in adrenal androgens between the ages of about 6–8 years.

2. Gonadarche: activation of gonadal sex steroid production occurring several years later.

The onset of puberty is characterized by an increase In frequency and amplitude of GNRH pulses, which stimulates LH and FSH secretion and hence gonadal adipose tissue secretes hormones, including leptin, and leptin appears to play a permissive role in puberty. Kisspeptin, released from hypothalamic neurons, stimulates GPR54 receptors on GNRH neurosecretory cells and increases GNRH secretion. Both leptin and kisspeptin are essential for puberty and attainment of fertility.

7.Cell:

47.Basic method of cell signaling are:
   a) Juxtacrine
   b) Paracrine
   c) Endocrine
   d) Autocrine
   e) All of above
      Answer: e

There are four basic methods of cell signalling:
• Juxtacrine
• Paracrine
• Endocrine
• Autocrine.
Each of these methods requires a signalling molecule and a cell surface receptor.
Depending on the type and location of the signalling molecules (also known as ligands) they can be categorized as hormones, cytokines, chemokines, or neurotransmitters.

48.Intracellular receptor required for:
   a) Steroid
   b) Thyroid
   c) Retinoid acid
   d) Vitamin D3
   e) All of above
      Answer: e

Receptors that are exclusively intracellular (necessitating the ligand to physically cross the cell membrane) include:
• Steroid hormone receptors
• Thyroid hormone receptors
• Retinoic acid receptors
• Vitamin D3 receptors.
Intracellular secondary messengers (where the ligand first interacts with a cell surface receptor) include:

- Calcium
- Nitric oxide
- Diacylglycerol
- Inositol triphosphate.

49. Molecule processed by endoplasmic reticulum transported out of cell by:
    a) Golgi appratus
    b) Lysosome
    c) Peroxisome
    d) Cytoskeleton
    e) All of above

    Answer: a

50. Manufacturing factory for protein is:
    a) Cytoplasm
    b) Endoplasmic reticulum
    c) Chaperons
    d) Golgi apparatus
    e) Ribosomes

    Answer: e

51. ATP produce in:
    a) Cytoplasm
    b) Endoplasmic reticulum
    c) Mitochondria
    d) Golgi apparatus
    e) Ribosomes

    Answer: e

52. Bacteria are digested in:
    a) Cytoplasm
    b) Endoplasmic reticulum
    c) Mitochondria
    d) Lysosomes
    e) Ribosomes

    Answer: d

What is a cell?

Cells are the basic building blocks of all living things. The human body is composed of trillions of cells. They provide structure for the body, take in nutrients from food, convert those nutrients into energy, and carry out specialized functions. Cells also contain the body's hereditary material and can make copies of themselves.

Cells have many parts, each with a different function. Some of these parts, called organelles, are specialized structures that perform certain tasks within the cell. Human cells contain the following major parts:

Cytoplasm

> Within cells, the cytoplasm is made up of a jelly-like fluid (called the cytosol) and other structures that surround the nucleus.

Cytoskeleton

> The cytoskeleton is a network of long fibers that make up the cell's structural framework. The cytoskeleton has several critical functions, including determining cell shape, participating in cell division, and allowing cells to move. It also provides a track-like system that directs the movement of organelles and other substances within cells.

Endoplasmic reticulum (ER)

> This organelle helps process molecules created by the cell. The endoplasmic reticulum also transports these molecules to their specific destinations either inside or outside the cell.

Golgi apparatus

> The Golgi apparatus packages molecules processed by the endoplasmic reticulum to be transported out of the cell.

Lysosomes and peroxisomes

> These organelles are the recycling center of the cell. They digest foreign bacteria that invade the cell, though away toxic substances, and recycle worn-out cell components.

Mitochondria

Mitochondria are complex organelles that convert energy from food into a form that the cell can use. They have their own genetic material, separate from the DNA in the nucleus, and can make copies of themselves.

Nucleus

The nucleus serves as the cell's command center, sending directions to the cell to grow, mature, divide, or die. It also houses DNA (deoxyribonucleic acid), the cell's hereditary material. The nucleus is surrounded by a membrane called the nuclear envelope, which protects the DNA and separates the nucleus from the rest of the cell.

Plasma membrane

The plasma membrane is the outer lining of the cell. It separates the cell from its environment and allows materials to enter and leave the cell.

Ribosomes

Ribosomes are organelles that process the cell's genetic instructions to create proteins. These organelles can float freely in the cytoplasm or be connected to the endoplasmic reticulum.

8.Microbilogy

1) Staphylococcus aureus
   a) Gram positive
   b) Pathogenic
   c) Coagulase positive
   d) Form yellow colony on culture
   e) All of above

Answer: e

2) Neisseria is:
   a) Gram negative
   b) Gram positive
   c) Strict anaerobes
   d) Form yellow colony on culture
   e) Bacilli

Answer: a

3) Process of taking free DNA from environment is called:
   a) Transduction
   b) Transformation
   c) Conjugation
   d) Plasmapherosis
   e) Organogenesis

Answer: b

4) Process of transfer of DNA from one bacteria to another with help of virus is called:
   a) Transduction
   b) Transformation
   c) Conjugation
   d) Plasmapherosis
   e) Organogenesis

Answer: a

5) Transfer of genetic material from one bacteria to another bacteria by forming sex pilus is called:
   a) Transduction
   b) Transformation
   c) Conjugation
   d) Plasmapherosis
   e) Organogenesis

Answer: c

Bacteria can exchange DNA and acquire (or lose) genes by varied means:

1. **Transformation:** many bacteria can take up freeDNA (released by dying organisms, not necessarily of the same species) from the extracellular environment.

2. **Transduction:** DNA can also be transferred from one bacterium to another by means of viruses thatInfect bacteria (bacteriophages).

3. **Conjugation:** Bacteria can exchange DNA directly(usually plasmids) by forming a long protein structure, the sex pilus, which binds two cells and allows aConjugal bridge to form, through which DNA can pass.This occurs most frequently with gram-negative

Organisms and allows genes coding for antibiotic resistance (for example) to spread rapidly.

6) Staphylococcus aureus:
   a) Cause cellulitis, boil and surgical site infection
   b) Toxic shock syndrome in tampon users
   c) Mrsa have mutation in penicillin binding protein
   d) Flucloxacillin is effective in beta-lactamase producing bacteria
   e) All of above

Answer: e

Staphylococci

● S. *Aureus* causes skin and soft tissue infections such as cellulitis, boils, and surgical wound infection, and it can also cause bacteraemia, endocarditis, and osteomyelitis.

• *S. Aureus* produces exotoxins, which can cause food poisoning, and also staphylococcal toxic shock syndrome, seen in tampon-users, where the vagina gets infected with *S. Aureus* and the toxin is absorbed systemically. • Most *S. Aureus* (> 90 %) are resistant to penicillin by means of beta-lactamase production, but can still be treated with flucloxacillin, which is not degraded by the beta- lactamase. Some *S. Aureus* have a mutant penicillin binding protein in the cell wall (PBP 2A), which renders it resistant to all beta-lactam antibiotics. This is referred to as methicillin-resistant *S. Aureus*, or MRSA. These organisms can still be treated with several other antibiotics, including vancomycin.

7) False statement about streptococci:

    a) Beta haemolytic streptococci cause partial haemolysis on blood agar

    b) Beta haemolytic streptococci classified according to carbohydrate present on outer cell surface

    c) Group B beta haemolytic streptococci i.e streptococcal algectasia is important cause of neonatal sepsis

    d) Streptococci sensitive to penicillin

    e) Some enterococci resistant to vancomycin also

Answer: a

Streptococci* and *enterococci

Streptococci and *enterococci* are gram-positive cocci that normally grow in chains, or sometimes pairs.

Classified as:

1) beta-haemolytic *streptococci* (which cause complete haemolysis of the red cells in the agar),

2) alpha-haemolytic *streptococci* (which cause partial lysis and thus green/brown discoloration of the agar), 3) gamma-haemolytic *streptococci* (which cause no lysis at all).

The alphahaemolytic *streptococci* are also known as viridans *streptococci*.

--beta-haemolytic *streptococci* are further categorized according to the particular sugar-compounds on their outer cell surface — the lancefield group.

Lancefield groups are often used interchangeably with species names. Thus, Group a beta-haemolytic *streptococci* are equivalent to *S. Pyogenes*, and group B beta-haemolytic *streptococci* equate to *S. Agalactiae* (a significant cause of neonatal sepsis).*Enterococci* were formerly known as 'faecal streps', being found in the gut, but they are genetically a separate group and belong to lancefield group D.

The *streptococci* are generally susceptible to penicillin or amoxicillin; *enterococci* tend to be more resistant, and some may even be resistant to vancomycin.

8) 40 years male HIV positive presented with brain abscess. Microscopy show gram positive, aerobic, weakly acid fast. Likely organism is:

a) Nocardia asteroid
b) Actinomyces
c) Stretptococci pyogens
d) Staphylococcus aureus
e) Enterococci

Answer: a

Nocardia,actinomyces
These are both branching gram-positive rods,
• *Nocardia* is aerobic, and is also (weakly) acid-fast (see '*mycobacteria*' section below). It is normally an environmental organism and tends to infect the immunocompromised or those with chronic lung disease. Typical diseases are brain abscess and persisting suppurative lung infection.
The most common species is *N. Asteroides.*

9) 40 years female having poor oral dentition presented with cervicofacial abscess and abdominal pain pus from lesion show non acid fast, anaerobic organism with sulphur granules. Likely organism is:

a) Nocardia asteroid
b) Actinomyces
c) Stretptococci pyogens
d) Staphylococcus aureus
e) Enterococci

Answer: b

• *Actinomyces* (commonest species: A. *Israelii*) are anaerobic, not acid-fast, and may colonize and infect the mouths of those with poor dentition. Infections are usually secondary to oral colonization and include cervicofacial abscesses, and aspiration or swallowing of organisms leading to thoracic, abdominal, and disseminated disease. Pus from these lesions often contains 'sulphur granules', which consist of a mycelial mass and may be up to a few mm in size.

10)   13 years male. Presented with pharyngitis. Microscopy show gram positive bacilli aerobic bacilli. Likely organism is:

a) Nocardia asteroid

b) Corynebacterium diphtheriae

c) Stretptococci pyogens

d) Staphylococcus aureus

e) Enterococci

Answer: b

Aerobic gram-positive bacilli

Corynebacteria are aerobic, **gram positive bacilli** and include *c. Diphtheriae*

This often carries a bacteriophage that codes for a potent exotoxin, which causes the illness diphtheria.

• The toxin is a classic subunit toxin: the beta-unit binds to host cells and the alpha-unit is released into the cytoplasm, where it switches off protein production leading to cell death.

• The illness begins as pharyngitis and the effects of the toxin are first seen in local upper airway tissues, and later in the heart and nervous tissue.

• A potent vaccine made from inactivated toxin so this illness is now very rare in the developed world.

11)   Gram positive aerobic bacilli responsible for preterm labour is:

a) Listeria monocytogen

b) Actinomyces

c) Stretptococci pyogens

d) Staphylococcus aureus

e) Enterococci

Answer: a

Listeria monocytogenes is widely distributed in the environment and is mainly a soil-dwelling aerobe, which can also be carried asymptomatically in the gastrointestinal tract of humans and many animal species.

• It can contaminate processed meats, dairy foods, and salads during preparation.

• It can grow at wide ranges of ph (5.6–9.6) and temperature (1–45 ° c), and thus can multiply in refrigerated food.

• The infection is usually harmless to healthy adults but it can cause meningitis in the immunocompromised and the elderly.

• In pregnancy it can cross the placenta to infect the fetus, resulting in miscarriage, preterm delivery, or term delivery of a baby with septicaemia or meningitis. Pregnant women are advised to avoid certain high-risk foods, pâté and soft cheeses in particular.

• Ampicillin is considered the drug of choice for treatment.

12)   Anthrax is caused by:
   a) Nocardia asteroid
   b) Actinomyces
   c) Stretptococci pyogens
   d) Staphylococcus aureus
   e) Bacillus anthracis

Answer: e

13)   Food poisoning because of reheated rice due to:
   a) Bacillus anthracis
   b) Bacillus cereus
   c) Stretptococci pyogens
   d) Staphylococcus aureus
   e) Enterococci

Answer: b

Bacillus spp. Are a large group of aerobic spore-forming environmental organisms, mostly harmless. Exceptions are *B. Cereus*, which can cause food poisoning (typically associated with reheated rice), and *B. Anthracis*, the cause of anthrax.

14)   Most common cause of urinary tract infection is. (clue: it is a gram negative rods, facultative anaerobic, ferment lactose):

a) Nocardia asteroid

b) Actinomyces

c) Stretptococci pyogens

d) Staphylococcus aureus

e) E. Coli

Answer: e

15)   Gram negative cocci which occur in pair isolated from endocervix of sexually active women likely organism is:

a) N. Gonorrhoeae

b) E. Coli

c) Stretptococci pyogens

d) Staphylococcus aureus

e) Bacillus anthracis

Answer: a

Neisseriae are aerobic gram-negative cocci, typically found in pairs; they grow best with added CO_2 and are oxidase positive. There are several species, distinguished by their use of different sugars; the two pathogenic species are *N. Meningitidis* and *N. Gonorrhoeae*.

• *N. Meningitidis* causes meningococcal sepsis and meningitis; it is spread by respiratory droplets and saliva.there are several serogroups based on capsular polysaccharide; A, B, and C are the most common, and a vaccine against serogroup C is now widely used in the UK. The organism remains penicillin sensitive and this is the agent of choice.

• *N. Gonorrhoeae* causes gonorrhoea, acute pelvic inflamatory disease, rarely septicaemia and septic arthritis, and ophthalmia neonatorum in babies born to mothers with active genital disease.

• The organism is fastidious, susceptible to drying out or cooling, and has complex nutritional requirements, needing special enriched media to grow.

• Spread is sexual, and the usual site of infections in females is the endocervix, and the urethra in males.

• Antibiotic resistance, particularly to penicillin and also quinolones, is common.

16)   Soft ulcer is caused by:
   a) Haemophilus influenzae
   b) Actinomyces
   c) Stretptococci pyogens
   d) Haemophilus ducreyi
   e) Bacillus anthracis

Answer: d

The main pathogenic species, *haemophilus influenzae*, is a small gram-negative rod. It is nutritionally fastidious, needing haemin (X-factor) and nicotinamide (V-factor) for growth;

• the other important *haemophilus* is *H. Ducreyi*, the causative agent of chancroid (soft ulcer).

17)   Gram positive spore forming anaerobic rod responsible for tetanus is
   a) Clostridium perfringes
   b) Clostridium botulinum
   c) Clostridium tetani
   d) Haemophilus ducreyi
   e) Bacillus anthracis

Answer: c

18)   Gram positive spore forming anaerobic rod responsible for food poisoning in canned food is:
   a) Clostridium perfringes
   b) Clostridium botulinum
   c) Clostridium tetani

d) Haemophilus ducreyi

e) Bacillus anthracis

Answer: b

19) Gram positive spore forming anaerobic rod responsibe for gas gangrene is:

a) Clostridium perfringes

b) Clostridium botulinum

c) Clostridium tetani

d) Haemophilus ducreyi

e) Bacillus anthracis

Answer: a

20) 25 years male presented with cough with sputum since 20 days not responding to antibiotics. Sputum examination show gram positive acid fast bacilli. Likely characteristic of bacilli is

a) It is mycobacterium tuberculosis

b) Ziehl neilson stain and auramine stain used for identification

c) Take several weaks for culture

d) Lowenstein-jensen media used for culture

e) All of above

Answer: e

21) Long slender coiled bacterium which cause yaw is

a) Treponema pallidum pallidum

b) Treponema pallidum pertenue

c) Treponema pallidum carateum

d) Haemophilus ducreyi

e) Bacillus anthracis

Answer: b

22) Long slender coiled bacterium which cause pinta is

a) Treponema pallidum pallidum

b) Treponema pallidum pertenue

c) Treponema pallidum carateum

d) Haemophilus ducreyi

e) Bacillus anthracis

Answer: c

23) Long slender coiled bacterium which cause syphilis is

a) Treponema pallidum pallidum

b) Treponema pallidum pertenue

c) Treponema pallidum carateum

d) Haemophilus ducreyi

e) Bacillus anthracis

Answer: a

24) Painless chancre is characteristic of

a) Primary syphilis

b) Secondary syphilis

c) Tertiary syphilis

d) Haemophilus ducreyi

e) Bacillus anthracis

Answer: a

Non-venereal syphilis, yaws (*T. Pallidum pertenue*), and pinta (*T. Carateum*).

• The organism cannot be cultured (except using animals, which is not practicable in a routine laboratory) and so serological tests are used for diagnosis.

Reagin tests: the level of reagin antibody correlates with disease activity. The classic reagin test is the 'venereal disease reference laboratory' test — the VDRL.

• Venereal syphilis has three stages:

1. *Primary syphilis* is marked by a painless ulcer (chancre) at the site of inoculation (usually genital); this then heals.

2. Some weeks later there is a generalized fever and rash, associated with systemic dissemination of the Treponemes throughout the body (*secondary syphilis*).

This resolves, but some patients go on to develop Latent syphilis.

3. After several years this latent syphilis presents as

Progressive vascular or neurological disease (*tertiary Syphilis*).

• Mothers with primary or latent infection may spread the infection haematogenously through the placenta to their babies, resulting in *congenital syphilis*. Affected babies may be stillborn, or survive but are born with the systemic (i.e. Secondary) phase of syphilis.

25)   Which of following is not feature of borrelia:
a) Borelia burgdorferi carried by ixodes tick
b) Cause lyme disease
c) Culture is difficult
d) Isolated bell`s palsy
e) All of above

Answer: e

Borrelia

• *B. Burgdorferi* is carried by *ixodes* ticks, which usually infect deer.

• Infection results in lyme disease, characterized by an initial rash at the site of the tick bite (erythema chronicum migrans) followed by chronic neurological or bone/joint problems; a common manifestation is isolated Bell's palsy.

• Culture of the organism is difficult and serology is used for diagnosis

26)   Organism with no cell wall and fried egg appearance on culture is:
a) Treponema pallidum pallidum
b) Treponema pallidum pertenue
c) Treponema pallidum carateum
d) Mycoplasma
e) Bacillus anthracis

Answer: d

27)   Most common cause of atypical pneumonia in young adult is:
a) Treponema pallidum pallidum
b) Treponema pallidum pertenue
c) Treponema pallidum carateum

d) Ureaplasma urealyticum

e) Mycoplasma

Answer: e

Mycoplasma

No cell wall- antibiotics that inhibit cell wall synthesis,

E.g. Penicillin and cephalosporin, will be ineffectiveIn *mycoplasma* infections.

Colonies are small and easily missed. Colonies are often glassy in appearance and may have an opaque central zone, giving rise to a 'fried egg' appearance.

• *M. Pneumoniae* causes 'atypical' pneumonia, it is the Most common cause of pneumonia in young adults.

• *Ureaplasma urealyticum* (characterized by the presence of a urease enzyme, allowing it to metabolize urea) has been implicated in respiratory and other infections of neonates.

28)   Q-fever caused by:

a) Coxiella burnetti

b) Treponema pallidum pertenue

c) Treponema pallidum carateum

d) Ureaplasma urealyticum

e) Mycoplasma

Answer: a

29)   Infectious form of chlamydia is:

a) Elementary body

b) Reticular body

c) Inclusion body

d) None of above

e) All of above

Answer: a

Chlamydia

These are obligate intracellular bacteria they cannot generate their own ATP

Exist in two forms: the elementary body is the smallInfective form taken up by a host cell; this then reorganizes into the reticulate body, which replicates and eventually fills the cell (giving rise to the inclusion body seen on microscopy). These then convert into elementary bodies and are released (or the cell lyses).

  30)   25 year sexually active women presented with increase frequency of micturition. Culture is non diagnostic. Likely organism is:
  a) Mycoplasma
  b) E. Coli
  c) N. Gonorrea
  d) Chlamydia
  e) Streptococci

Answer: d

 Genital infections are spread sexually and are frequently asymptomatic, which facilitates onward transmission. They include urethritis (men), cervicitis, and occasionally pelvic inflammatory disease, which can lead to scarring of the uterus or fallopian tubes, with risk of infertility, miscarriage, or ectopic pregnancy (women). • *chlamydia* cannot be grown on solid media. Cell culture is possible but difficult, and diagnosis is usually by enzyme immunoassay detection of antigen, or (more recently) by Amplification of nucleic acid, which has the advantage of being able to use urine rather than cervical or urethral swabs.

  31)   Most common cause of viral encephalitis is:
  a) HSV i
  b) HSV ii
  c) Cytomegalovirus
  d) Epstein bar virus
  e) Varicella zoster virus

Answer: a

  32)   Shingle`s caused by:
  a) HSV I
  b) Reactivation of varicella zoster virus
  c) Cytomegalovirus
  d) Epstein bar virus

e) Varicella zoster virus

Answer: b

33)   25 years primigravida had fever malaise headache in mid trimester. On birth her child has fever, jaundice, pneumonia, thrombocytopenia. Most likely diagnosis is:
a) HSV i
b) HSV ii
c) Cytomegalovirus
d) Epstein bar virus
e) Varicella zoster virus

Answer: c

Herpes viruses
-Enveloped DNA
Latent for many years in nerve ganglia (herpes simplex, varicella-zoster) or lymphocytes (cytomegalovirus, epstein-barr virus).

Herpes simplex i and ii
HSV-i usually affects the mouth or face and is spread by oral or salivary contact; most people have a primary infection in childhood. Latent infection can re-emerge as cold sores of the lips, sometimes triggered by various stimuli: cold, sunlight, and other infections. HSV-i is also the most common cause of viral encephalitis.

HSV-ii affects the genital area and is spread by sexual contact. It can also lead to recurring painful genital lesions. Childbirth during a primary HSV-ii infection can lead to severe generalized neonatal infection.

Varicella-zoster virus (VZV)
This causes chickenpox in the non-immune. Latent infection can re-emerge as shingles (localized vesicular skin lesions, in the region of a single dermatome). Nearly all adults are immune.

Infection in pregnancy may be associated with severe disease and pneumonitis; rarely, the fetus may be infected *in utero* and suffer reactivation leading to scarring and limb hypoplasia.

Cytomegalovirus (CMV)

This causes an acute illness with fever, malaise, headache, and sometimes mild hepatitis. Latency occurs in blood mononuclear cells and can re-emerge in immunocompromised patients (including HIV) to cause a variety of syndromes, including retinitis and colitis. The virus is found in blood and body fluids, and spread occurs at birth, from breast milk, from direct contact with other children, and later on through sexual contact. Primary infection of a pregnant Mother may lead to severe congenital infection of the Infant, with growth restriction, fever, jaundice, pneumonitis, and thrombocytopenia.

34)   Which of following virus transmitted by faeco-oral rout

   a) Hepatitis a
   b) Hepatitis b
   c) Hepatitis c
   d) Hepatitis d
   e) All of above

Answer: a
Hepatitis a virus- RNA virus
Spread via the faeco-oral route. No chronic infection or carriage of the virus, and infection confers lifelong immunity.Effective vaccines are available;Diagnosis is by detection of IgM in serum.

35)   False statement about hepatitis b virus infection is:

   a) Sexually transmitted
   b) HBsAg and HBeAg suggest active infection with high viral load
   c) RNA virus
   d) Vaccine contain anti-HBsAB antibody
   e) Anti-HBcAb antibody persist for life

Answer: c
Hepatitis b virus (HBV)
Enveloped DNA virus (the rest are RNA viruses). Blood and body fluids contain the virus (not faeces) and spread is via blood and sexual contact, or vertically during childbirth.

Subclinical infection seen Chronic infection cause chronic hepatitis, cirrhosis, and hepatocellular cancer.

• Surface antigen (HBsAg) refers to envelope proteins; HbsAg in the blood suggests an active infection but does not indicate whether the virus can be passed to others .antibodies to HBsAg indicate previous exposure to hepatitis B virus, but the virus is no longer present and the person cannot pass on the virus to others. This antibody provides lifelong immunity from HBV infection

• Core antigen (HBcAg) is the capsid protein but disappears early in the course of infection. Antibodies to the core antigen are produced during an acute HBV infection and afterwards. They are present in chronic HBV *carriers* as well as in those who have cleared the virus, and usually persist for life. Their presence implies a past infection at some time, as this antigen is absent from the vaccine.

• The e-antigen is a protein contained within the capsid; its presence in the blood implies that a large number of infectious virus particles are present, and thus a high level of infectivity. Conversely, the presence of antibody to the e-antigen, even in the presence of HBsAg, implies low-level infectivity.

• Hepatitis B vaccine should be given to those at high risk of infection, for example family or sexual contacts of cases, healthcare workers, and babies born to carrier status and infectious mothers (these babies should also be given hepatitis B immune globulin).

HbsAg(-) Total anti-HBc(-) Anti-HBs(-)	Susceptible
HbsAg(-) Total anti-HBc(+) Anti-HBs(+)	Immune due to natural infection
HbsAg(-) Total anti-HBc(-) Anti-HBs(+)	Immune due to hepatitis B vaccination
HbsAg(+) Total anti-HBc(+) IgM anti-HBc(+) Anti-HBs(-)	Acutely infected
HbsAg(+) Total anti-HBc(+) IgM anti-HBc(-) Anti-HBs(-)	Chronically infected
HbsAg(-) Total anti-HBc(+) Anti-HBc(-)	Four possibilities: 1) Resolved infections 2) False positive thus susceptible 3) Low level chronic infection 4) Resolving infection

36)   A school teacher 23 years 19 week pregnant come for routine anamoly scan . In scan fetus had hydrops. She gave history of slapped-cheeks disease in one of her student. Likely virus is

a) HSV i
b) Parvovirus b19
c) Cytomegalovirus
d) Epstein bar virus
e) Varicella zoster virus

Answer: b

Parvovirus b19 is the only human pathogenic parvovirus; it causes erythema infectiousum in children (also known as 'fifth disease', or 'slapped-cheeks disease').

- It is the only single-stranded dna virus.
- It is spread by the respiratory route.

The virus infects red cell precursors(attach on P antigen), and may precipitate an aplastic crisis in patients who already have chronic haemolytic anaemia.

- Infection in pregnancy may result in fetal infection, with anaemia and hydrops — but most infections in pregnancy have no ill effect on the fetus.

37) Most common single defect of congenital rubella syndrome is:
a) Cataract and glaucoma
b) PDA
c) Sensorineural deafness
d) Neonatal purpura
e) Hepatosplenomegaly

Answer: c

Rubella virus — an enveloped RNA virus of the togavirus group — causes rubella or German measles.

- The congenital rubella syndrome includes deafness, cataracts or retinopathy, mental retardation, microcephaly, and cardiac abnormalities. The illness is prevented by the MMR vaccine, but cases are still seen in the unvaccinated.

38) Characteristic of Rubeola are:
a) Koplik's spot on oral mucosa
b) Pneumonia most common cause of death
c) Rarely cause subacute sclerosing panencephalitis
d) Erythematous and maculopapular rash spread from face to periphery
e) All of above

Answer: e

Measles (rubeola)

• This is the most infectious of the exanthems. Koplik's spots may develop on the oral mucosa — these resemble grains of salt or sand.

• The rash is erythematous and maculopapular, and spreads from face to trunk to extremities.

• Pneumonia is common and accounts for most of the deaths. Acute encephalitis is rare, and very rarely childhood infection is followed by subacute sclerosing panencephalitis (SSPE), which leads to progressive and irreversible dementia.

39)   False statement among following is:
   a) Gradual change in influenza a genome is called antigenic drift
   b) Gradual change in influenza a genome is called antigenic shift
   c) Pandemic caused by antigenic shift
   d) Croup is caused by para influenza virus
   e) Common cold cause by rhinovirus

Answer: b

Influenza virus

This consists of a coiled RNA nucleocapsid within a lipid envelope containing neuraminidase (N) and haemaglutinin (H) glycoproteins. There are three types: influenza a is found in humans and animals (including pigs and birds), B and C infect humans only and cause milder illness. Incidence is seasonal, with winter epidemics.

• Continual mutations of the influenza A genome lead to gradual changes in the surface antigens (antigenic drift) allowing a degree of immune evasion and contributing to the yearly epidemics.

• More dramatic antigenic changes (antigenic shift) occur rarely, leading to effectively new viruses; this can result in global pandemics.

Respiratory syncytial virus (RSV) is the major cause of bronchiolitis in young children.

• **Parainfluenza virus** causes laryngotracheobronchitis (croup).

- **Rhinovirus**, which is related to the enteroviruses, is the main cause of the common cold.

    40)   Commonest cause of gastroenteritis in infant is:

    a) Enterovirus

    b) Norovirus

    c) Rotavirus

    d) Epstein bar virus

    e) Varicella zoster virus

Answer: c

Rotavirus is an RNA virus with a double-layered capsid, giving it a characteristic wheel-like appearance on electron microscopy. It is the commonest cause of gastroenteritis in infants and young children.

    41)   Which of following is not characteristic of hiv virus:

    a) RNA retrovirus

    b) Bind to GP41 on CD 8 T cell

    c) Transmitted by infected blood , sexual contact, breast feeding

    d) Viral DNA which produce from RNA get incorporated into host DNA and produce number of copies of viruses

    e) If HIV RNA load is <50 copies per ml then patient can be counseled for vaginal delivery

Answer: b

HIV – retrovirus: The virus binds via an envelope glycoprotein, GP41, to the CD4 molecule on the surface of T lymphocytes.

- The viral RNA enters the cell and is transcribed into DNA by the reverse transcriptase. The viral DNA is then incorporated into the host genome, and serves as a template for further virus production.

- Spread is either sexual, by infected blood, during childbirth, or by breastfeeding.

    42)   False statement about HPV is:

    a) DNA virus

b) Butcher`s wart is caused by type 7

c) 6,11,16,18 cause anogenital wart

d) 16, 18 cause wart of hand and feet

e) 16,18,31, 33 causative agent for carcinoma of cervix

Answer: d

Human papillomaviruses (HPV — wart viruses) are DNA viruses that specifically infect skin and mucous membrane cells.

Types 1, 2, 3, and 4 cause warts of the hands and feet; type 7 causes butcher's warts (common warts in people who regularly handle raw meat, poultry, and fish),

Types 6, 11, 16, and 18 cause anogenital warts

Type 16,18,31,33 known as high risk group responsible for carcinoma of cervix.

43)   Charectoristic of candida albicans are:

a) Form germ tube in culture

b) Causative agent for oral thrush

c) Common cause of vaginal infection in diabetes patient

d) Cultured on saboured agar

e) All of above

Answer: e

Candida albicans is typically distinguished in the laboratory by its ability to form a 'germ tube' — a single hypha — when cultured in serum.

• Oral *candida* infection (oral thrush) can occur in otherwise healthy adults, but may be a marker for immunosuppression; HIV patients may get severe oral and oesophageal *candida* infections.

• *candida* is a common cause of vaginal infection and discharge (which is typically creamy-white); this is more common in diabetes, in pregnancy, and following antibiotic use, but many infections occur without any of these factors.

44)   Charectoristic of Entamoeba hystolytica are:

a) Causative agent for amoebic dysentery

b) Cyst form is spherical with four nuclei

c) It can cause liver abscess

d) Treatment of choice is metronidazole

e) All of above

Answer: e

Entamoeba histolytica

• This is an intestinal amoeba, the cause of amoebic dysentery.

• It has a cyst form that is spherical with four nuclei, averaging 10–15 microns in diameter, and a motile amoeboid trophozoite form that is larger (up to 40 microns) with a single nucleus.

E. Histolytica may spread via the portal veins and cause an amoebic liver abscess, which can present months or years after the episode of dysentery.

• Diagnosis depends on the clinical presentation; acute dysentery is best diagnosed by examining a fresh sample (a 'hot stool') for trophozoites, which may contain ingested red cells. Older samples rarely contain visible trophozoites, but cysts may be seen.

• In amoebic liver abscess, cysts may be absent from the faeces, and serology is more definitive in the diagnosis. Aspiration of the cyst should be avoided, for fear of peritoneal seeding of amoebae.

• treatment of both amoebic dysentery and liver abscess is with metronidazole, followed by diloxanide furoate to eradicate organisms within the gut.

45)   Commonest parasite found in UK is:

a) Entamoeba histolytica

b) Cryptosporidium parvum

c) Gardia lamblia

d) Plasmodium

e) Leishmania

Answer: b

Cryptosporidium parvum

• This is the commonest parasitic infection reported in the uk; it may arise from livestock animals or other humans.

• like *giardia*, it may be spread via contaminated drinking water.

• The cysts are small (2.5 microns) and easily overlooked — they can be detected using modified acid-fast stains.

• Paromomycin was formerly used to treat severe infections seen in aids patients; more recently nitazoxanide has been licensed in the usa (but not yet in the uk) for treatment.

46)   Infective form of plasmodium is :
    a) Sporozoitis
    b) Merozoitis
    c) Female gamete
    d) Male gamete
    e) All of above

Answer: a

47)   Temperature used in steam autoclaving is:
    a) 135 degree celsius for 3 minute
    b) 125 degree celsius for 3 minute
    c) 135 degree celsius for 15 minute
    d) 130 degree celsius for 3 minute
    e) 130 degree celsius for 15 minute

Answer: a

48)   Which of following is killed vaccine:
    a) Polio
    b) Hepatitis A
    c) Cholera
    d) Rabies
    e) All of above

Answer: e

49)   Which of following is live vaccine:
    a) Mumps
    b) Measles
    c) Rubella
    d) Yellow fever
    e) All of above

Answer: e

Important questins:

1. Target for beta lactam antibiotics is:
   a) Penicillin binding protein
   b) N acetyl glucosamine
   c) N acetyl muramic acid
   d) Teichoic acid
   e) Beta lacamase in peri plasmic space
   Answer: a

2. False statement among following is:
   a) Plasmid code for antibiotic resistant
   b) Pasmid code for sugar fermentation
   c) Bacteria can transfer antibiotic resistance through plasmid
   d) Mycoplasma have rigid cell wall
   e) Chlamydiae lack peptidoglycans
   Answer: d

3. Which of the following is aerobic gram positive cocci:
   a) *Stphyloccocus aureus*
   b) *Peptostreptococci*
   c) *Bacillus species*
   d) *Neisseria gonorrhea*
   e) *Vibrio cholera*
   Answer: a

4. Wrong statement among following is:
   a) Specimen for culture should be taken before treatment start
   b) Specimen should be kept for 4 ^{0}c and transported to laboratory
   c) Chlamydiae and virus survive better at -70^{0}c
   d) Gonococcus should be directly plated bedside or rapidly transported to laboratory

e) To increase likelihood of positive result swab stick dipped in pus is always preferred than liquid pus

Answer: e

5. Which of the following commensals present in vaginal flora responsible for acidic ph:
   a) Lactobacilli
   b) Diphtheroid
   c) Staphylococci
   d) Alpha haemolytic streptococci
   e) Actinomyces

   Answer: a

6. False statement regarding listeria monocytogen is :
   a) Infection occure in late pregnancy
   b) One of the organism responsible for preterm labour
   c) Miliary granuloma with focal necrosis is common lesion found in post partum examination of placenta
   d) Intrapartum infection will lead to predominantly meningitis in neonate with incubation period of 5 to 7 days
   e) Colonize intrauterine devices

   Answer: e

7. Which of the following is not a feature of vaginosis:
   a) Presence of clue cells
   b) Fishy smell
   c) Presence of vaginal wall gland infection
   d) Watery vaginal discharge
   e) Ph > 5.0

   Answer: c

8. False statement among the following is:
   a) Mycoplasma hominis is found in 20% of sexually active women
   b) Ureaplasma urealyticum found in 80% of sexually active women

    c) Mycoplasma should be consider as cause of post partum pyrexia and treatment with tetracyclin should be consider if fever not settle down.

    d) Chlamydia can be cultured in artificial media

    e) N. Gonorrhoeae commonly infect columnar epithelium cells

    Answer: d

9. Antibiotics acting on cell wall are:

    a) Penicillin

    b) Cephalosporins

    c) Monobactams and carbapenems

    d) Vancomycin & teicoplanin

    e) All of the above

    Answer: e

10. Antibiotics acting on ribosomes are:

    a) Erthromycin

    b) Clindamycin

    c) Tetracyclin

    d) Amynoglycoside

    e) All of the above

    Answer: e

11. Antibiotic resistance is not mediated by:

    a) Antibiotics may not get into cell

    b) Rapidly eliminatedby efflux mechanism

    c) Enzyme may destroy antibiotics

    d) Target site may get altered

    e) None of above

    Answer: e

12. Antisepsis was first demonstrated by:

    a) Josep lister

    b) Berkeley moyhnihan

    c) Robert koch

    d) Lou paster

    e) Edward jenner

    Answer: a

13. Srerilization is defined as not a single organism in
    a) One million surgical packs
    b) One lakh surgical packs
    c) Ten thousand surgical packs
    d) Thousand surgical packs
    e) Hundred surgical packs
    Answer: a

14. false statement among following is:
    a) Basic time temperature use in UK for pure steam autoclaving is 134-137°c for 3 min.
    b) In downward displacement autoclave instruments are packed loosely
    c) Cetrimde is commonly used against P. Aeruginosa in laboratory
    d) For processing of endoscope mechanical washer should be used
    e) Ethelene oxide is used to sterilize heat sensitive devices
    Answer: c

15. Primigravida 34 weeks with gestatinal diabetes mellitus presented with curdy white vaginal discharge with formation of pseudohyphae in culture and formation of germ tube in serum, organism can be:
    a) Cryptococcus neoformans
    b) Candida albicans
    c) Histoplasma capsulatum
    d) Trichophyton
    e) Microsporum
    Answer: b

16. 30 years old sexually active women presented with purulent vaginal discharge, itching, ph> 5.0. On wet mount preparation organism with of size of white blood cell with flagella present. Probable organism is :

a) Candida albicans
b) T. Vaginalis
c) T. Gondi
d) G. Lamblia
e) Cyptococcus
   Answer: b

17. Indications for delivery in case of corona virus infection are:
    a) Maternal rapid deterioration
    b) Failure to maintain adequate ventilation
    c) Multi organ failure
    d) Difficulty in mechanical ventilation due to gravid uterus
    e) All of above

18. Incidence of rubella infection in fetus of women with rubella infection upto 12 week of gestation is :
    a) 54%
    b) 80%
    c) 25%
    d) 15%
    e) 40%
       Answer: b

19. Parvovirus B19 bind to globoside (P antigen) present on
    a) RBC
    b) WBC
    c) Platelets
    d) Lymphocyte
    e) Nerve cells
       Answer: a

20. Chances of transmission of HIV 1 infection from mother to fetus in absence of antiretroviral treatment and with treatment and caesarean section is

a) 50% & 20%
b) 80% & 20%
c) 15% & 2%
d) 30% & 2%
e) 2% & 30%
   Answer: c

21. Wrong statement regarding hepatitis b virus infection is :
    a) Infant delivered of HBsAg and HBeAg positive should be given vaccine and HBIg
    b) Infant delivered of HBsAg and anti- HBe positive should be given vaccine without HBIg
    c) Infant delivered of HBsAg and HBeAg status not known should be given vaccine and HBIg
    d) DNA virus
    e) Transmitted by contaminated water
       Answer: e

22. HPV high risk group include
    a) 6
    b) 11
    c) 16
    d) 18
    e) 31 and both c and d

Answer: e

9.Pathology

1. Most common type of collagen is:
   a) Type 1
   b) Type 2
   c) Type 3
   d) Type 4
   e) Type 5

Answer: a

2. Type of collagen found in basement membrane is:
   a) Type 1
   b) Type 2
   c) Type 3
   d) Type 4
   e) Type 5

Answer: d

Types of collagen
1. Type 1 is the most common, has the highest tensile Strength, and is found everywhere in the body including bones, skin, tendons, and in most organs.
2. Type 2 collagen is found in cartilage and vitreous humour only.
3. Type 3 is found in granulation tissue, embryonic tissue, the uterus, and in keloids.
4. Type 4 collagen is found in basement membranes.

3. Glanzmann thromboasthenia is due to:
   a) VwF
   b) GpIb
   c) Gp2b3a
   d) Autoantibodies against platelet
   e) All of above

Answer: c

4. Characteristic of thrombotic thrombocytopenic purpura is:
   a) Thrombocytopenia
   b) Prolonged bleeding time
   c) Normal PT, APTT
   d) Fragmented cells in peripheral smear
   e) All of above

Answer: e

Immune thrombocytopenic purpura (ITP)
•Autoantibodies produced against own platelets, which coat the platelets.
• The IgG-coated platelets are destroyed in the spleen
Leading to thrombocytopenia.
Two forms of ITP:
1. *Acute form*, usually a self-limiting illness seen in children after a viral illness.
2. *Chronic form*, usually in women of reproductive age and commonly associated with lupus. May present with nose bleeds, menorrhagia, and ecchymosis.

Thrombotic thrombocytopenic purpura (TTP)
• Due to generalized and widespread platelet thrombi formation (not true thrombi but fibrin and platelets stuck together).
• Characteristically there is no activation of the coagulation system.
• Usually affects adult females.
• There is a clinical pentad of fever, thrombocytopenia, Microangiopathic haemolytic anaemia, neurological Symptoms, and renal failure.
• Lab findings include thrombocytopenia, prolonged bleeding time, normal coagulation (PT and PTT) test, fragmented red blood cells, and schistocytes on blood film.

5. As compared to TTP , HUS has
   a) More renal problems
   b) No thrombocytopenia
   c) More neurological problems

d) Increase PT

e) Increase APTT

Answer: c

Haemolytic uraemic syndrome (HUS)

• On the opposite end of the disease spectrum to TTP.

• The same pentad of signs and symptoms is involved.

• TTP has more neurologic symptoms; HUS has more Renal problems.

• TTP is usually found in adults, HUS usually in children, and they are associated with bloody diarrhoea after infection from *e. Coli*, 0157h.

6. Features of haemophilia a is:

a) Because of factor VIII deficiency

b) Haemarthrosis

c) Easy bleeding

d) Increase PTT is the only findings

e) All of above

Answer: d

Haemophilia A (VIII deficiency)

• An x-linked recessive disorder and therefore affects Males.

• Haemarthrosis, easy bleeding following trauma.

• Single abnormality is raised PTT

• Treatment is factor VIII replacement.

Thrombophilia b (IX deficiency)

• Also an x-linked disorder.

• Clinically identical to haemophilia A.

• Distinction made by factor VIII and IX assays.

7. Which of following is not feature of DIC :

a) Reduced platelet

b) Increase PT and PTT

c) Reduce fibrinogen

d) Increase FDP

e) Increase fibrinogen

Answer: e

Disseminated intravascular coagulopathy (DIC)

• Always secondary to another disease, e.g. Abruption, malignancy, leukaemia, or infection (particularly gramnegative sepsis).

• There is generalized formation of thrombi, which uses up all the platelets, coagulation factors, and fi brinogen in a consumptive coagulopathy leading to excessive bleeding.

• Diagnosis requires the presence of four conditions:

1. Reduced platelet count
2. Increased PT and PTT
3. Reduced fibrinogen
4. Increased fibrinogen degradation products (or d-dimers).

• Treatment — treat the underlying cause and correct the coagulopathy.

8. Major stages of shock are:
   a) Compensated
   b) Decompensated
   c) Irreversible
   d) None of above
   e) All of above

Answer: e

Three major stages of shock

1. Compensatory stage — perfusion to the vital organs is maintained by reflex mechanisms including catecholamine release and activation of the sympathetic and reninangiotensin systems (RAS).

2. Decompensated stage — reduced tissue perfusion resulting in reversible cellular injury, metabolic acidosis, and electrolyte disturbances.

3. Irreversible stage — organ failure and death even if the original injury is removed.

9. Features of down syndrome is:
   a) 95% because of non-disjunction
   b) Trisomy 21
   c) Increased frequency of leukaemia

d) Increase incidence of hirschsprung's disease

e) All of above

Answer: e

Down syndrome, 21 chromosome trisomy 95 % secondary to non-disjunction, 4 % RobertsonianTranslocation features include flat face, low nasal bridge, wide-set eyes, short broad neck, low-set ears, speckled appearance of the iris (brush field spots), single simian crease in the hand, cardiac defects including ASD, VSD, duodenal atresia (double bubble sign on ultrasound scan), and Hirschsprung's disease.

■ 15 to 25 % have increased risk of leukaemia, particularly acute lymphocytic leukaemia

■ Alzheimer's disease (amyloid protein deposition in the brain from the extra chromosome 21) by ≥ 40Years of age.

10. Edward syndrome features are:

a) Trisomy 18

b) Severe mental retardation

c) Low set ear

d) Micrognathia

e) All of above

Answer: e

● *Edward syndrome:*

■ Trisomy 18, 46 xx/xy + 18

Features include severe mental retardation, low-set ears, overlapping flexed fingers, micrognathia, rockerbottom feet (from excessive connective tissue at the base of the foot), and death soon after birth (severe malformations).

● *Patau syndrome:*

Trisomy 13, 47 XX/XY + 13 non-disjunction

Features include severe mental retardation, microcephaly, extra digits, cleft lip and palate, chromosomal deletions (e.g. 46 XY/XY 5p–), and VSD.

11. Wrong statement about Klinefelter's syndrome:

a) 47 XXY/48XXXY

b) Male with hypogonadism, atrophic testes, infertility, gynaecomastia

c) Meiotic disjuction

d) High pitch voice

e) No production of testosteron

Answer: c

12. Features of turner's syndrome is:

a) 45 XO

b) Infertile female

c) Short stature

d) Coaractation of aorta

e) All of above

Answer: e

Klinefelter's syndrome:

47 XXY/48XXXY

A meiotic chromosomal non-disjunction disorder

Results in male hypogonadism, atrophic, fibrotic testes, no production of testosterone, infertility, high-pitched voice, gynaecomastia.

● *Turner's syndrome:*

45 XO

Female hypogonadism (two X chromosomes required for normal ovarian development), the ovaries are streaked (by the fibrous tissue bands)

Primary amenorrhoea, reduced oestrogen, short stature, failure of secondary sex characteristics, cystic Hygromas (dilated lymphatic channels underneath the skin, which eventually leave redundant skin around the neck), aortic coarctation, hydrops fetalis, may be stillborn.

13. False statement among following is:

a) Mutation of both allele required in autosomal recessive disease

b) Phenylketonuria is due to defect in enzyme phenylalanine hydroxylase

c) Cystic fibrosis is because of defect in chloride channels , genes for which present on chromosome no 7 at 508 position

d) In phenylketonuria give phenylalanine containing diet

e) Male with cystic fibrosis associated with congenital absence of vas deferance

Answer:d

Autosomal recessive disorders

●General characteristics:

Early in onset, presenting early in infancy or childhood,complete penetrance (i.e. Likely to express if Inherited),Tends to involve enzyme proteins, e.g. Cystic fibrosis, alkaptonuria, albinism, glycogen storage disease.Mutation of both alleles required.

●*Phenylketonuria (PKU):*

Autosomal recessive disorder

Defect in the enzyme phenylalanine hydroxylase leading to accumulation of toxic levels of phenylalanine in the brain

Light-coloured skin and hair

Treatment is dietary restriction of phenylalanine.

● Cystic fibrosis (CF):

The defect is in the CF-transmembrane conductance

Regulator, a chloride channel protein responsible for

Anion transport.The gene is on chromosome 7 and the deletion is at position 508 in 70 % of cases

There is production of viscid mucus, which blocks the ducts in organs, e.g. In the lung leading to pneumonia and bronchiectasis, and in the gut leading to meconium ileus. Other features include pancreatic atrophy and fibrosis, and congenital absence of the Vas deferens.

14.False statement about familial hypercholesterolaemia is:

a) Autosomal dominant disorder

b) Defect in IDL receptor gene

c) LDL cholesterol level incrases

d) Present in 1 in 1000 individual

e) Xanthoma and premature atherosclerosis are features of disease

Answer:d

Familial hypercholesterolaemia:

Most common inherited disorder (affecting 1 in 500)

Defect is a mutation in the IDL receptor gene

No functional IDL receptors in the liver, thereforeLDL-cholesterol levels increase, and the liver responds by producing even more cholesterol, because of lack of negative feedback no inhibition of HMGCoA reductase, which exacerbates the process.

May be heterozygous or homozygous

Xanthomas (lipid-laden macrophages) and premature artherosclerosis.

15. False statement about Marfan`s syndrome is:

a) Because of defect in fibrillin gene
b) Short individual with long arm, leg, and fingers
c) Bilateral subluxation of lens
d) Hyperextensibility of joints
e) Aortic dissection

Answer: b

Marfan's syndrome:

Defect is in the fibrillin gene (a glycoprotein that functions as a scaffold protein and helps to align elastin fibres)

Affects skeletal systems

Affected individuals are tall with long arms, legs, bones, and fingers .

Hyperextensible joints and chest wall deformities.

Bilateral subluxation of the lens, aortic dissection from cystic medial necrosis leading to aneurysms, aortic insufficiency and mitral valve prolapse

16. Patient is presented with cafe-au-let spot, pheochromocytoma, pigmented iris. Likely diagnosis:

a) Marfan` syndrome
b) Neurofibromatosis i

c) Down`s syndrome

d) Ehler`s danlos syndrome

e) Cystic fibrosis

Answer: b

Neurofibromatosis (Von Recklinghausen's disease) types 1 and 2:

Approximately 90 % of cases are type 1.

Mutation is in neurofibroma NF1 tumour suppressor gene on chromosome 17, responsible for producing Neurofibromin.

Patient presents with café-au-lait spots, nerve bundle, and branch lesions, increased risk of pheochromocytoma and meningiomas,pigmented iris

Type 2 — 10 % of cases

Mutation in tumour suppressor gene type 2 on chromosome 22

Gene product is merlin but its function is unknown.

17. Which of following is x linked disorder:

   a) Fragile x syndrome

   b) Engelman`s syndrome

   c) Prader willi syndrome

   d) Huntington`s disease

   e) All of above

Answer: e

18. Atopy and asthma is :

   a) Type i hypersensitivity reaction

   b) Type ii hypersensitivity reaction

   c) Type iii hypersensitivity reaction

   d) Type iv hypersensitivity reaction

   e) None of above

Answer: a

19. Grave`s disease, myasthenia gravis, good pasture are

   a) Type i hypersensitivity reaction

   b) Type ii hypersensitivity reaction

   c) Type iii hypersensitivity reaction

d) Type iv hypersensitivity reaction

e) None of above

Answer: b

20.Lupus and rheumatoid arthritis

a) Type i hypersensitivity reaction

b) Type ii hypersensitivity reaction

c) Type iii hypersensitivity reaction

d) Type iv hypersensitivity reaction

e) None of above

Answer: c

21.SLE is charectorised by:

a) Affect women more than men

b) Anti-dsDNA is more specific than anti-SM antibodies

c) Associated with congenital heart block in fetus

d) Characterized by malar rashes, lymphopenia, thrombocytopenia

e) All of above

Answer: e

● Systemic lupus erythematosus (SLE):

A chronic autoimmune disease characterized by loss of self-tolerance and production of lots of autoantibodies

Affects women more than men, usually reproductive age women, and Africans more than Caucasians.

Due to autoantibodies against nuclear proteins including histones, DNA, and other RNA proteins.

Antinuclear antibodies (ANA) are commonly raised, but they are not specific. Specific antibodies for SLE are anti-dsDNA (double-stranded DNA), and anti-SM antibodies (aka anti-Smith); anti-DNA is the more sensitive of the two.Tissue injury in SLE is usually a combination of types 2 and 3 hypersensitivity reaction; that is antibody targeted against specific tissue and deposition of immune complexes.

Diseases include anaemia, thrombocytopenia, arthritis, neutropenia, lymphopenia, malar skin rash, diffuse glomerulonephritis and membranous glomerulonephritis leading to nephrotic syndrome, endocarditis, and pericarditis.Treatment   is   with   steroids   and immunosuppressants.

22. A patient of rheumatoid arthritis presented with dryness of eye and dryness of mouth, with positive SSA & SSB antibodies, likely diagnosis is:
    a) SLE
    b) Sjogren`s syndrome
    c) Scleroderma
    d) BTK mutation
    e) Di george`s syndrome

Answer: b

23. Patient is presented with thick claw like fingers, dysphagia, dyspnea with positive anti-DNA topoisomerase. Likely diagnosis is:
    a) Diffuse scleroderma
    b) Localize scleroderma
    c) Sjogren`s syndrome
    d) SLE
    e) Rheumatoid arthritis

Answer: a

24. Patient is presented calcinosis , raynaud` phenomeonon, oesophageal dysmotility, sclerodactyly, telangectsia, positive anticentromere antibody likely diagnosis is:
    a) Diffuse scleroderma
    b) Localize scleroderma
    c) Sjogren`s syndrome
    d) SLE
    e) Rheumatoid arthritis

Answer: b

Diffused scleroderma is associated with anti-DNA topoisomerase-1 antibodies and affects approximately 70 % Of cases; there is widespread involvement of the hands and face leading to thick and fibrotic claw-like fingers, and also involvement of the internal organs including. The oesophagus (dysphagia), gastrointestinal tract (malabsorption), lungs (fibrosis, dyspneoa), heart (arrhythmias), and kidneys (renal failure)

Localized (form) scleroderma (aka the CREST syndrome):
C — Calcinosis, R — Raynaud's phenomenon, E— Oesophageal dysmotility, S— Sclerodactyly, T— Telangiectasia. It is associated with anti-centromereAntibodies involving the skin, hands, and face, leading to clawed hands and smooth, tight face; it may also involve the internal organs later in its course. The localized form has a more benign prognosis compared to the systemic form.

25. Immunodeficiency syndrome are:
    a) X- linked agammaglobulinemia
    b) Di-george syndrome
    c) SCID
    d) Wiskott Aldrich syndrome
    e) All of above

Answer: e

26. Which of following is wrong about amyloidosis:
    a) It is a beta pleated structure which give bright red color on congo red staining and aple green birefringence under polarized light
    b) Multiple myloma and B cell lymphoma are example of primary amyloidosis where there is deposition of light chain.
    c) Reactive systemic amyloidosis is characterized by deposition of SAA. E.g. Tuberculosis and Crohn`s disease
    d) In familial mediterranean fever deposition of al
    e) A-beta 2 macroglobulin deposited in hemodialysis associated amyloidosis

Answer: d

Amyloidosis
- Amyloid is deposited in a very specific configuration Called a ' bet-pleated sheet'.
- It is eosinophilic pink under the microscope.
- It gives a bright red/pink colour when stained with congo red and because of its beta-pleated sheet the congo red also produces another effect when placed under polarized light — 'apple green birefringence' (i.e. Some areas will have green and others yellowish colouration).

Systemic forms of amyloidosis:

1. Primary amyloidosis
- Usually caused by plasma cell malignancy including multiple myloma and b-cell lymphoma.
- The protein deposited as amyloid is the light chain called AL type (amyloid-light chain).

2. Reactive systemic amyloidosis (secondary amyloidosis)
- The fibrillar protein is called serum amyloid a (SAA), which is an acute phase reactant protein produced by the liver.
- This type of amyloidosis occurs in inflammatory states such as tuberculosis, rheumatoid arthritis, SLE, Crohn's disease, ulcerative colitis, and longstanding osteomyelitis, and it is the underlying inflammatory disease that stimulates the liver production of SAA.

3. Familial mediterranean fever (inherited amyloidosis)
- Autosomal recessive disorder.
- Also produced by SAA protein.
- Characterized by recurrent bouts of infections, fever, and neutrophil dysfunction.

4. Haemodialysis-associated amyloidosis
- Usually diagnosed on dialysed patients; the dialyzing membrane is not very good at handling and filtering proteins, especially A-Beta2 macroglobulin, which accumulates and deposits in tissues, especially in the wrists where it may cause carpal tunnel syndrome.
- The amyloid protein is called A-Beta-2 macroglobulin.
- The protein accumulated is Beta-2 macroglobulin.

Localized forms of amyloidosis

Senile cerebral amyloidosis (Alzheimer's disease)
- The amyloid protein is A-beta

• The fibrillar protein is called beta-amyloid precursor protein (BAPP).
• The gene for BAPP is located on chromosome 21, which is why down syndrome patients with an extra chromosome 21 get Alzheimer's disease.
• The amyloid is found in the centre of all amyloid plaques and also within the cerebral vessels.
Senile cardiac amyloidosis
• Usually in older men over 70 years of age and may result in heart failure.
• Restrictive cardiomyopathy.
Endocrine organs and tumour amyloidosis
• For example, medullary carcinoma of the thyroid, which is a c-cell tumour producing calcitonin.
• The tumour is surrounded by deposits of pro-calcitonin, which forms beta-pleated sheets resulting in amyloid.
• Prognosis is very poor.

27. Which of following pair is wrong:
    a) Alpha fetoprotein- yolk sac tumor
    b) Beta HCG -choriocarcinoma
    c) Calcitonin-thyroid follicular cells
    d) CEA- colon carcinoma
    e) Ca-125 -epithelial ovarian tumors

Answer: c

Tumour markers include:
• Alpha-feto protein (AFP) — hepatomas and yolk sac tumours
• Beta-HCG — trophoblastic tumours and choriocarcinomas
• Calcitonin — thyroid c-cells
• Carcino-embryonic antigen (CEA) — lung, pancreas, Breast, and colon
• Ca 125 — epithelial ovarian tumours
• Ca19–9 — important for pancreatic cancers
• Placental alkaline phosphatase — seminomas
• PSA and prostatic acid phosphotase — prostate cancer

28. Which of following is wrong about polyarthritis nodosa:
    a) Due to segmental necrotizing vasculitis

b) Medium size arteries usually involved
c) 75% cases have antibodies against own neutrophil
d) Lung most commonly involved
e) Associated with hepatitis B infection

Answer: d

Polyarthritis nodosa:
Due to segmental necrotizing vasculitis
Sequelae include thrombosis, weakened vessels, and aneurysms.Any organ may be involved except the lungs. Medium-sized arteries are usually involved, including kidneys, heart, gastrointestinal system, and muscles .there is a low-grade fever, malaise, and weight loss. 30 % of cases are associated with infection, e.g. Hepatitis B virus.Autoantibodies against own neutrophils (specifically against neutrophil peroxidise) are present in 75 % of cases a variant of polyarthritis nodosa displays vasculitis with granulomas and eosinophilia.

29. 35 years female patient is presented with sinusitis pneumonia, nasal ulceration and acute glomerulonephritis, likely diagnosis is:
a) Wegner`s granulomatosis
b) Polyarthritis nodosa
c) Kawasaki`s disease
d) Giant cell arteritis
e) Henoch shonlen purpura

Answer: a

Wegener's granulomatosis:
A rare necrotizing vasculitis with granuloma formation
Usually in the age group of 40–60 years.
Affects the nose, lungs, sinuses, and kidneys resulting in pneumonia, sinusitis, nasal Ulceration, and dominant renal disease, with cause of death usually acute glomerulonephritis nephritis.
Microscopy reveals fibrinoid necrosis and granulomas ■ autoantibodies against neutrophils present in 93 % of cases.If

untreated (usually with cyclophosphamide) mortality is 80 % within a year.

30. 65 years female patient is presented with malaise, weight loss, fever, throbbing headache, facial pain, visual disturbances. Increase in ESR. Likely diagnosis is:
   a) Wegner`s granulomatosis
   b) Polyarthritis nodosa
   c) Kawasaki`s disease
   d) Giant cell arteritis
   e) Henoch shonlen purpura

Answer: d

Temporal (giant cell) arteritis:
This is the most common form of arteritis and usually Occurs in the elderly
Associated with HLA DR4 small and medium-sized arteries involved, particularly the facial artery; the aortic arch may be involved including the cranial branches
Patients present with throbbing headaches, visual disturbances facial pains, fever, malaise, weight loss, and nodularity of arteries.
The ESR is raised and there is formation of granulomas with segmental multi-nucleated giant cells.
Treatment is with steroid with typically a good response.

31. 45 years female patient is presented absence radial pulse in both arm, BP normal , likely diagnosis is:
   a) Wegner`s granulomatosis
   b) Polyarthritis nodosa
   c) Kawasaki`s disease
   d) Giant cell arteritis
   e) Takayasu arteritis

Answer: e

Takayasu arteritis (pulscless disease):

Agranulomatous arteritis with loss of the pulse from The thickening intima of the vessels

Affects the aortic arch and its branches.

Usually involves young Asian women.

Response to steroid is variable.

32. 45 years male smoker presented with pain in leg on walking. Likely diagnosis is:
   a) Wegner`s granulomatosis
   b) Thromboangitis obliterans
   c) Kawasaki`s disease
   d) Giant cell arteritis
   e) Takayasu arteritis

Answer: b

Thromboangitis obliterans (buerger's disease):

Affects young male smokers

Involves the extremities

Vessel lumen obliterated by inflammatory thrombi

Patient may present with gangrene or claudication

Treatment is to stop smoking.

33. 2 year child presented with fever, maculopapular rashes not responding to treatment. Likely diagnosis is:
   a) Wegner`s granulomatosis
   b) Polyarthritis nodosa
   c) Kawasaki`s disease
   d) Giant cell arteritis
   e) Takayasu arteritis

Answer: c

Kawasaki disease:

Affects children <4 years of age.

Common in Hawaii and Japan.

There is an acute febrile illness, conjunctivitis, lymphadenopathy, fever, maculopapular skin rash.

Coronary artery involvement in 70 % of cases with thrombosis or aneurysm in 1 to 2 % of patients.

Disease is self-limiting and is thought to be due to a virus.

34. 40 years african women presented with fever, malaise,night sweat . X ray show bilateral hilar lymphadenopathy, tissue biopsy show non caeseating granuloma, blood sample show increase ace. Likely diagnosis is:

   a) Wegner`s granulomatosis
   b) Polyarthritis nodosa
   c) Kawasaki`s disease
   d) Sarcoidosis
   e) Tuberculosis

Answer: d

35. Newborn male delivered by LSCS at 30 week of gestation presented with difficulty in respiratory difficulty. X- ray show ground glass appearance likely diagnosis is:

   a) Acute respiratory distress syndrome
   b) Hyaline membrane disease
   c) Polycystic kidney
   d) Giant cell arteritis
   e) Takayasu arteritis

Answer: b

Newborn respiratory distress syndrome (RDS, hyaline membrane disease)
- Associated with prematurity.
- 60 % of neonates <28 weeks will suffer from rds.
- Associated with elective caesarean section, diabetes Mellitus, and multiple births.
- Due to the deficiency of pulmonary surfactant.
- The infants are usually normal at birth, followed by rapid onset of respiratory insufficiency.
- Chest x-ray reveals ground glass appearance.

• Microscopic findings are identical to ARDS.

• Treatment is with surfactant, oxygen, and ventilation.

• Mortality is as high as 30 % .

• Long-term sequelae include bronchopulmonary dysplasia, pulmonary hypertension, and increased pulmonary arterial pressure.

36. 8 years male child presented with haematuria, urine examination show RBC cast. Had history of sore throat 6 month back. Tissue biopsy show, epithelial hump immunofluorescence show IgM, IgG & complement c deposition throughout glomeruli, likely diagnosis is:
   a) Acute glomerulonephritis
   b) Polyarteritis nodosa
   c) Urinary tract infection
   d) Polycystic disease of kidney
   e) IgA nephropathy

Answer: a

37. Young male with hematuria and hemoptysis, with presence of autoantibodies against type iv collagen basement membrane of lung and glomeruli, likely diagnosis is:
   a) Acute glomerulonephritis
   b) Polyarteritis nodosa
   c) Goodpasture`s disease(type ii hypersensitivity reaction)
   d) Polycystic disease of kidney
   e) IgA nephropathy

Answer: c

38. Most common form of nephritis characterized by deposition of IgA in mesengial cells is called
   a) Acute glomerulonephritis
   b) Polyarteritis nodosa
   c) Goodpasture`s disease
   d) Polycystic disease of kidney

e) IgA nephropathy (Berger`s disease)

Answer: e

39. Wrong statement about adult polycystic kidney disease is:

a) Autosomal dominant

b) Defect in polycystin-I gene present on chromosome 17

c) Presented in 40 years of age with hypertension, and renal insufficiency

d) Pancreatic cyst, hepatic cyst, Berry`s aneurysm , mitral valve prolapse may be associated with it.

e) Autosomal recessive

Answer: e

40. False statement among following is:

a) Crohn`s disease usually affect from mouth to anus

b) Terminal ileum is most common side of crohn`s disease

c) Crohn`s disease have transmural inflammation , non caseating granuloma and skip lesion

d) Crohn`s disease associated with HLA B27

e) Pseudo polyp present in ulcerative colitis

Answer: d

Crohn's disease (regional enteritis)

●Usually affects caucasian women, peak age 10–30 years and 50–60 years.

● Less common than ulcerative colitis.

● There is usually fever, peritoneal fistulas, and malabsorption if the terminal ileum is involved.

●May affect any part of the gastrointestinal system from the mouth to the anus, but the terminal ileum is the more common site.

Diagnosis is made by endoscopy, which shows skip areas (lesions) and strictures, and by biopsy, which shows transmural inflammation, non-caseating granulomas, and strictures.

- Unlike ulcerative colitis there are not many extra-intestinal manifestations.
- About 1–3 % may progress to carcinoma.

Ulcerative colitis

- Associated with HLA B27.
- Always involves the rectum from where it spreads proximally, usually to the large intestine, and rarely to the ileum.
- There is extensive mucosal ulceration and formation of pseudopolyps (areas that have not ulcerated and therefore stand out like polyps); there are no strictures.
- Microscopy shows inflammation limited to the mucosal and the submucosal layers, and crypt abscesses.
- Complications include toxic megacolon and a 5–25 % risk of colonic cancer.
- Extra-intestinal manifestations— primary sclerosing cholangitis.

41. Conjunctivitis , urethritis , arthritis is feature of:
    a) Reiter`s disease
    b) Multiple endocrine neoplasm syndrome
    c) Ducchenne`s muscular dystrophy
    d) Ankylosing spondylitis
    e) IgA nephropathy (Berger`s disease)

Answer: a

42. Defect in dystrophin gene cause
    a) Reiter`s disease
    b) Multiple endocrine neoplasm syndrome
    c) Ducchenne`s muscular dystrophy
    d) Ankylosing spondylitis
    e) IgA nephropathy (Berger`s disease)

Answer: c

Important questions:

1. Increase in number of cells in tissue called:
   a) Hypoplasia

b) Atrophy

c) Hypertrophy

d) Heperplasia

e) Metaplasia

Answer: d

2. Carcinoma of cervix most commonly occur at:

a) Ectocervix

b) Endocervix

c) Transformation zone

d) Same at all above places

e) None of above

Answer: c

3. Commonest cause of first and early second trimester miscarriage is :

a) Chromosomal abnormality

b) Infection

c) Smoking

d) Maternal diseases

e) Alcoholism

Answer: a

4. wrong statement among following is:

a) Complete hydatidiform mole is diploid

b) Incomplete hydatidiform mole is triploid

c) Possibility of developing in persistent trophoblastic neoplasm in complete and incomplete hydatidiform mole is 15% and 0.5% respectively

d) No need of serum hcg measurement in follow up of molar pregnancy

e) Molar pregnancy may follow live birth.

Answer: d

5. Sequence means

a) Any deviation from structure, form and function

b) Abnormal organization of tissue

c) Abnormality in the shape or position of part of body due to mechanical forces
d) Multiple abnormality derived from single presumed prior factor
e) Multiple associated abnormalities thought to be pathogenically related but not representing sequence
   Answer: d

11.Pharmacology:

1. Mifepristone, misoprostol dinaprostone are :
   a) Progesterone ,oxytocin, PGE1 receptor antagonist respectively
   b) Progesterone receptor antagonist PGE1 receptor agonist, PGE 2 agonist respectively
   c) PGE 2 agonist , PGE1 agonist , progesterone agonist respectively
   d) PGE1 , PGE2 agonist ,progesterone receptor agonist respectively
   e) Progesterone , PGE1 and PGE2 antagonist respectively

Answer: b

2) Atosiban is:
   a) Oxytocin receptor blocker
   b) Progesterone antagonist
   c) Use as tocolytic
   d) Both a and c
   e) Progesterone agonist

Answer: a

3) Patient should avoid pregnancy for period of _____before/after high doses of vitamin K :
   a) 1month/1 year
   b) 2 month/2 year
   c) 1month/2 year
   d) 2month/1 year
   e) 3month/1 year

Answer: c

4) Warfarin act by
   a) Inhibition of factor vii
   b) Inhibition of factor x
   c) Inhibition of factor vii

d) Inhibition of reduction of vitamin K oxide form

e) Inhibition of factor xii

Answer: d

5) After starting Warfarin there is thrombosis in superficial vein. This is due to:

a) Inhibition of factor VII

b) Inhibition of factor X

c) Inhibition of factor VII

d) Inhibition of reduction of vitamin K oxide form

e) Inhibition of protein C and S before inhibition of reductase enzyme

Answer: e

6) After starting Warfarin there is thrombosis in superficial vein. This effect can be prevented by:

a) Giving Vitamin K before warferin

b) Giving acecoumarin before warferin

c) Giving heparin before warferin

d) Giving protein C and S before warferin

e) Giving FFP before warferin

Answer: C

7) Warfarin act in:

a) 6 hour

b) 12 hour

c) 18 hour

d) 12 days

e) 18 days

Answer: b

8) If patient is predispose to thrombosis INR should be maintain in between:

a) 2 to 4

b) 1 to 2

c) 4 to 8

d) 8 to 12

e) 12

Answer: a

Warfarin

Warfarin is an analogue of vitamin K, which competitively inhibits its reduction by competing for the active site of the reductase enzyme that reduces vitamin K oxide back to vitamin K.

Because of the slow production of the reduced form, Proteins C and S may be inhibited before other factors initially. As a result of the loss of these activated proteins, which normally inhibit coagulation by inactivating factors VIIA and VA, an anomalous reduction in INR and increase in intravascular coagulation may result.

Heparin may be given before warfarin to prevent these effects. An INR between 2 and 4 is desirable where patients are predisposed to thrombosis or its consequences. • Warfarin is rapidly absorbed and peak plasma concentrations are achieved within an hour, the effects on clotting take 12 hours to develop and last 4–5 days. • Warfarin is teratogenic during the first trimester of pregnancy and is also contraindicated in later pregnancy because of the danger of fetal intracranial haemorrhage. It passes into the breast milk in small amounts and may theoretically cause increased bleeding tendencies in the infant. Administration of vitamin K reduces this risk.

• Necrosis of breast or buttock caused by intravascular thrombosis of small vessels due to inhibition of protein c and, with overdose, haemorrhage may occur. Other oral anticoagulants are phenindione and acenocoumarol.

9) Heparin act by

a) Inhibition of antithrombin III

b) Activate antithrombin III

c) Inhibition of factor VII

d) Inhibition of reduction of vitamin K oxide form

e) Inhibition of factor XII

Answer: b

   10)   Half of life of heparin is:
   a) 1 day
   b) 2 days
   c) 1 hour
   d) 2 hour
   e) 1 week

Answer: c

   11)   Heparin induced thrombocytopenia due to antibody against heparin occur in:
   a) 1 day
   b) 2 days
   c) 5 days
   d) 2 hour
   e) 4 week

Answer: c

   12)   Hemorrhage due to heparin can be reversed by:
   a) Protamine
   b) Vitamin K
   c) Factor VII
   d) Normal saline
   e) Danaparoid

Answer: a

Heparin
● Heparin activates antithrombin III produced by the endothelium, which inhibits the action of thrombin (factor IIa) and factors IXa, Xa, XIa, and XII.
● Heparin is administered intravenously or subcutaneously and has a half life of about 1 hour. APTT is monitored.
● LMWH have a longer half life and zero-order elimination so their effects are more predictable.
● Heparins are large molecules and do not cross the placenta; however, they should be discontinued before delivery.
● The main side effect is haemorrhage, which can be treated by ceasing administration and, if necessary, administration of

protamine, which is less good at reversing the actions of LMWH.

• Heparin-induced thrombocytopenia may occur due to the development of antibodies after 4–5 days administration, and osteoporosis with much longer periods of treatment.

13) Primigravida 30 week 3 days started on antihypertensinve methyldopa 1 month back. Now she complaint of edema on both legs. What are side effects of methyldopa:
a) Sedation
b) Reduced libido
c) Edema
d) Post partum depression
e) All of above

Answer: e

14) Primigravida 30 week 3 days started on antihypertensinve 1 month back. Now her hemoglobin is 8 gm%. And comb's test positive. What is likely antihypertensive:
a) Ace inhibitors
b) Labetolol
c) Methyldopa
d) Nifedepine
e) Hydrilazine

Answer: c

15) Side effect because of which clonidine is not used today is:
a) Sedation
b) Reduced libido
c) Rebound hypertension
d) Post partum depression
e) All of above

Answer: c

Methyldopa is a prodrug, which is metabolized to its active metabolite alpha-methyl noradrenaline. Alpha-methyl noradrenaline that preferentially activates central alpha-2-receptors, thereby reducing sympathetic outflow and vasomotor tone. The delay in the onset of action of methyldopa observed clinically is in part due to the time required to convert methyldopa to its active metabolite.

There are, however, central side effects including sedation, drowsiness, dizziness, and reducedLibido because of its primary site of action.

Other side effects include oedema and positive coombs test. Clonidine is associated with severe rebound hypertension if discontinued abruptly and is rarely used in clinical practice. It also causes drowsiness and dry mouth.

16)　　Labetalol is:
   a) Selective beta1 blocker
   b) Selective beta2 blocker
   c) Non selective beta blocker
   d) Alpha blocker
   e) Direct vasodialator

Answer: c

17)　　Characteristics of labetalol are:
   a) Reduces myocardial oxygen demand and prevent reflex tachycardia
   b) Block Beta2 receptor at juxtraglomerular apparatus and thus prevent sodium and water retension.
   c) Should be avoided in asthmatic diabetic and peripheral vascular disease
   d) Can cause neonatal hypoglycemia
   e) All of above

Answer: e

Labetalol is a non-selective beta-blocker and it also exhibits additional alpha-blocking action.

●It exerts its antihypertensive effect mainly through blockade of the Beta1 receptors expressed in the heart. It reduces myocardial contractility, heart rate, cardiac output, myocardial oxygen demand, and blood pressure. It is not associated with orthostatic hypotension but there may be atrioventricular block and congestive cardiac failure.

The action of labetalol on the heart prevents reflex tachycardia following a drop in blood pressure. It opposes renin release through blockade of Beta2 effect in the juxtaglomerular apparatus; thus there is no sodium and water retention.

●Beta 2 receptors are expressed in the bronchioles, pancreas, and peripheral skeletal muscle vasculature. For this reason labetalol should be avoided in asthmatics, diabetics, and in people with peripheral vascular disease where beta receptor blockade may lead to bronchospasm, hypoglycaemia, or ischemic limb respectively.

Fetal effects include growth dysregulation with prolonged use. There may be neonatal hypoglycaemia and therapy should be discontinued gradually. Central effects include depression, fatigue, and sexual dysfunction.

18)   Which of following statement is wrong about nifedipine
   a) Belongs to dihydropiridine
   b) Block l type of calcium channels
   c) Good antihypertensive in black and old people
   d) Can cause bradycardia
   e) Can cause myocardial infarction

Answer: d

Nifedipine is the prototype of a class of vascular selective calcium channel antagonists known as the 'Dihydropyridines'. Nifedipine causes a marked vasodilatation in the hypertensive patient. This elicits a compensatory reflex tachycardia, which may be sufficiently severe to induce cardiac arrhythmias, myocardial infarction, and/or sudden death. This is particularly important in patients with underlying cardiac impairment.

The coronary arteries are perfused during the diastolic phase of the cardiac cycle. Therefore, during tachycardia the time available for the perfusion of the coronaries may be significantly reduced, with deleterious effects on the myocardium.

19)   Exacerbation of SLE is caused by:
   a) Hydralazine
   b) Nifedipine
   c) ACE inhibitor
   d) Labetalol
   e) Methyldopa

Answer: a

20)   Hydralazine is:
   a) Direct vasodilator
   b) ACE inhibitor
   c) Calcium channel blocker
   d) Non selective beta blocker
   e) Central alpha 2 blocker

Answer: a

Hydralazine:
• Hydralazine exerts vasodilatory effects by acting directly on the vasculature. It increases the release of endothelial derived relaxation factor (EDRF) i.e. Nitric oxide, a potent vasodilator.
The potent vasodilatation of cerebral vessels leads to headaches, whilst dilatation of other vascular beds elicits flushing and compensatory tachycardia, sweating, and fluid retention.
Hydralazine is metabolized by N-acetyltransferase, so it may accumulate in people with systemic lupus erythematosus and in slow acetylators. Main role in obstetrics is as a rapidly acting antihypertensive for severe hypertension and pre-eclampsia.

21)   Hyperkalemia is because of:

a) Hydralazine

b) Nifedipine

c) ACE inhibitor

d) Labetalol

e) Methyldopa

Answer: c

The accumulation of bradykinin following the use ofACE inhibitors is believed to be responsible for the dry cough observed in a third of patients on ACE Inhibitors, and also angioedema, which is found more commonly in black patients compared to their caucasian counterparts.Other side effects include hypotension, hypovolaemia, hyperkalaemia, and acute renal failure.

22)   Which of following compound is having strong anti-tusive action and no analgesic and no respiratory depression :

a) Morphine

b) Codeine

c) Pholcodine

d) Tramadol

e) Methyldopa

Answer: c

Morphine produces a powerful feeling of contentment and wellbeing.

Codeine does not produce euphoria.

Nalorphine produces dysphoria.

Morphine and other opiates cause respiratory depression. This is mediated by a decrease in the sensitivity of respiratory centre to PCO2.

Morphine is antitussive. This property does not correlate with analgesia or respiratory depression. Codeine is antitussive at sub-analgesic doses. Pholcodine is a modified opiate that has strong antitussive effects but little or no analgesia.

23)   Which of following compound is having strong anti-motility action and no analgesic and no respiratory depression, so used for diarrhea :

a) Morphine
b) Codeine
c) Pholcodine
d) Tramadol
e) Loperamide

Answer: e

Constipation. Loperamide, which is unable to cross the blood-brain barrier and so does not cause analgesia or respiratory depression, is widely used to treat diarrhoea.

24)   Which of following is not effect of Morphin:

a) Tolerance develop to vomiting
b) Tolerance develop to miosis
c) Tolerance not develop to constipation
d) Morphin withdrawl can cause yawning, diarrhea, shivering
e) Morphine release histamine from mass cells

Answer: b

Morphine can cause nausea and vomiting on first administration, due to an action on the chemoreceptor trigger zone in the medulla. This effect is usually transient and disappears on repeat administration.

Morphine causes pin-point pupils. This is centrally mediated and is an important diagnostic aid in opiate overdose.

Morphine (but not other opiates) releases histamine from mast cells. This can result in itching, urticaria, hypotension, and bronchoconstriction.

Tolerance occurs when a drug is administered repeatedly and the dose has to be increased to maintain the desired effect. Tolerance may occur with most opiate effects including analgesia and respiratory depression, but not with miosis or constipation.

Dependence is where adaptive changes have taken place in response to repeated administration of drugs and are most clearly seen as a withdrawal syndrome when the drug is withheld or its pharmacological action blocked. Opiate withdrawal comprises physical and psychological effects. Physical effects include abdominal cramps, diarrhoea, shivering, yawning, goose bumps, anxiety, and convulsions. Psychological effects are manifest as intense craving. Physical effects typically start within 12 hours, peak between 24–72 hours, and may last up to 14 days.

Psychological effects typically last much longer, sometimes years.

25) Local anesthetic drug act by:
   a) Blockage of potassium channel
   b) Blockage of sodium channel
   c) Blockage of calcium channel
   d) Opening of sodium channel
   e) Opening of potassium channel

Answer: b

LA block the generation and propagation of action potentials by blocking the Na + channels responsible for the upstroke of the action potential

26) Prilocaine and Benzocaine is not used in obstetrics practice because of:
   a) It cause hypotension
   b) Hypoglycemia in newborn
   c) Hyperglycemia in newborn
   d) Methaemoglobinaemia in newborn
   e) Hypocalcaemia in newborn

Answer: b
Prilocaine and benzocaine can induce methaemoglobinaemia and should not be used in obstetric procedures or in neonates

Important questins:

1. Drug which bind to Alpha1 glycoprotein is:
   a) Salicylates
   b) Warfarin
   c) NSAIDS

d) Beta-blocker

e) All of above

Answer: d

2. Microsomal enzyme inhibitor is:

a) Progestogen

b) Rifampicin

c) Theophyllin

d) Estrogen

e) Ehanol

Answer: d

3. Physiological changes in pregnancy that affect drug metabolism:

a) Distribution of all drugs increases

b) Delayed gastric emptying cause slow peak level of readily absorbable drug and increase bioavailability of slowly absorbable drug

c) Decrease albumin and raised free acid leads to increase level of albumin bind drugs

d) Enhance alveolar and intramascular drug absorption

e) All of above

Answer: e

4. Drugs used for tocolysis are

a) Beta $_2$ agonist

b) NSAIDS

c) Magnesium sulfate

d) A and b only

e) A,b,c

Answer: e

5. False statement regarding methyldopa is :

a) It is a prodrug

b) It readily cross placenta and achieve similar concentration in fetus as in mother

c) In 7.5 years of follow up children did not show any adverse effect

d) It can cause hemolytic anemia , thrombocytopenia, granulocytopenia , hypoprolactinaemia

e) It is metabolized to alpha-methyl-noradrenalin

Answer: d

6. Hydralazine :
   a) causes contraction of arteriolar smooth muscle
   b) It cause increase in vascular resistance to cerebral, coronary, and renal circulation.
   c) It does not cause postural hypotension
   d) Bradycardia is one of the side effect
   e) Lupus like syndrome in both mother and fetu

Answer: c

7. False statement regarding nifedepine:
   a) Dihydropyridine compound which act on fast voltage gated calcium channels and no effect on slow channels
   b) Cause tachycardia
   c) Last for 6 hours
   d) Used for induction of preterm labour
   e) Used should be limited to second and third trimester ideally

   Answer: d

8. False statement about oxytocin is:
   a) Octapeptide
   b) Synthesize in in paraventricular nucleus of hypothalamus
   c) Half life is 30 min
   d) 30 fold increase in oxytocin receptor at term
   e) High dose bolus can produce reflex hypotension and tachycardia

   Answer: c

9. Side effect of beta-agonist used during preterm labor

a) Tachycardia

b) Hypotension

c) Hypoglycemia

d) Hypokalemia

e) All of above

Answer: e

10. Mechanism of action of magnesium is

a) Decreases presynaptic glutamine release

b) Block NMDA receptor

c) Potentiation of adenosine action

d) Mitochondrial buffering and blockage of entry via voltage-gated channels

e) All above

Answer: e

11. Respiratory depression is common in neonates if Pethidine is used within hour of delivery

a) 3 hour

b) 6 hour

c) 10 hour

d) 13 hour

e) 16 hour

Answer : a

12. Drug use for treatment of SLE in pregnancy:

a) Methotrexate

b) Chlorambucil

c) Cyclophosphamide

d) Azathioprine

e) Isotretinoin

Answer: d

13. About use of anticoagulant in preganancy:

a) Warfarin interfere with vitamin a dependant coagulation factors(ii,vii,ix,x)

b) Warfarin cause chondrmalacia punctata

c) Heparin in glycosaminoglycans which act by inhibiting factor ii

d) Heparin crosses placenta

e) Non immune heparin associated thrombocytopenia occurs 3 to 4 week after therapy

Answer: b

14. Patient on anticonvulsant:

a) Sodium valproate and carbamazepine cause neural tube defect and spina bifida

b) If the women is convulsion free , there is usually no need to measure serum level of anticonvulsant drug

c) Vitamin K should be given in last 4 weeks of preganancy

d) Carbamazepine, phenytoin, and valproic acid are safe in preganancy

e) All of above

Answer: e

15. NSAIDS :

a) Do not cross placenta as it is albumin bind

b) Used to prevent neonatal haemorrhage

c) Leads to polyhydroamnios in pregnancy

d) Premature ductus closure and oligohydroamnios because of NSAIDS are reversible

e) Can be used till term

Answer: d

16. Which of the following drug when given within three month of conception in either of parent increases frequency of trisomy 21

a) Penicillin

b) Colchicine

c) Quinolones

d) Amynoglycosides

e) Chloramphenicol

Answer: b

17. Tetracycline cause:
    a) Arthropathy and phototoxicity in children
    b) Ototoxicity and renal toxicity
    c) Tooth disclouration
    d) Grey baby syndrome
    e) Idiosyncratic bone marrow depression
    Answer: c

18. Which of the following drug can cause hemolytic anaemia , hyperbillirubinaemia and kernicterus in neonate if given in third trimester of pregancancy:
    a) Sulfonamides
    b) Erythromycin
    c) Metronidazole
    d) Quinolones
    e) Tetracyclin
    Answer: a

19. False statement about trimethoprim :
    a) Readily cross placenta
    b) Inhibitor of dihydrofolate reductase
    c) Decrease serum homocystein concentration
    d) Tube defect
    e) Megaloblastic anaemia
    Answer: c

20. Acyclovir
    a) Inhibit viral RNA synthesis
    b) Converted acyclovir triphosphate by viral thymidine kinase
    c) Acyclovir triphosphate act as chain initiator
    d) Oral bioavaibility is good
    e) Not secreted in breast milk
    Answer: b

21. Triazole acts by:
    a) Inhibition of cytochrome p450
    b) Inhibition of sterol demethylase
    c) Prevent utilization of PABA for synthesis of folic acid

    d) Formation of highly reactive nitro anions

    e) Inhibit dihydrofolate reductase

    Answer: b

22. Anamoly cause by triazole is :

    a) Premature closure of petant ductus arteriosus

    b) Aplasia cutis

    c) Phacomalia

    d) Telepis equine varies

    e) Antley-Bixler syndrome

    Answer: e

23. Correct statement among following is:

    a) Thioamides act by preventing iodination of tyrosin residue

    b) Thioamides(propylthiouracil thiamazole, carbimazole) does not cross placenta

    c) High dose cause fetal hyperthyroidism

    d) Patient who are on maintenance dose of carbimazole need to be switch to propylthiouracil in preganancy

    e) Thioamides are contraindicated in breast feeding

    Answer: a

24. After taking more than 20mg of prednisolone how , breast feeding should be delayed for:

    a) No need of delay

    b) 40 minute

    c) 4 hour

    d) 40 hour

    e) 4 days

    Answer:c

25. Betamethasone administration for lung maturity in preterm baby associated with:

    a) Decrease incidence of respiratory distress syndrome

    b) Periventricular leukomalacia and intraventricular haemorrhage

    c) Hyperglaycemia

d) May precipitate myasthenia gravis and hypertensive crisis in mother

e) All of above

Answer: e

26. In order to avoid bladder toxicity Ifosfimide should be given with
   a) Chlorambusil
   b) Melphan
   c) Mesana
   d) Cyclophosphamide
   e) Dacarbazine

   Answer: c

27. Mechanism of action of alpha Cisplatin is:
   a) Inhibition of dihydrofolate reductase
   b) Purine analogue
   c) Intercalated between base pair and hinder DNA synthesis
   d) Form intra stand and interstand cross link
   e) Bind with tubulin and cause metaphase arrest

   Answer: d

28. Mechanism of action of combined oral contraceptive pill is:
   a) Progesterone act on hypothalamus to inhibit GNRH pulses and on pituitary to inhibit the oestrogen induced LH surge
   b) Oestrogen decrease the pituitary response to GNRH and follicular phase inhibit the FSH surge.
   c) Oestrogen and progesterone alter the transport of sperm, egg and fertilized ovum due to their effect on fallopian tube
   d) Progesterone cause thickening of cervical mucus
   e) All of the above

   Answer: e

29. Wrong statement about mechanism of action of progesterone only pills
    a) Blockade of ovulation due to slowing of GNRH pulse generator in 90 to 100% of cases
    b) Prevention of LH surge in 60-80% of cases
    c) Thickening of cervical mucus
    d) Alternation of intra-uterine environment
    e) None of above
       Answer: a

30. Which of the following is not effect of combined oral contraceptive pills:
    a) Increase the risk of infarction/stroke in smokers
    b) Decrease antithrombin iii and plasminogen activator
    c) Long term use associated with increase incidence of gall bladder disease
    d) Combined pill cause endometrial and ovarian cancer
    e) Slight increase in hepatic adenoma

    Answer: d

31. Patient taking oral contraceptive is a known case of tuberculosis. Which drug can cause contraceptive failure:
    a) Rifampicin
    b) Isoniazide
    c) Pyrazinamide
    d) Ethambutol
    e) Streptomycin
       Answer: a

12.Physiology

1. True statement among following is:
   a) Cardiac muscle have unstable resting membrane potential
   b) Short plateau phase
   c) Cardiac muscle cannot be tetanized
   d) Action potential transfer from one cell to another because of tight junction
   e) Voltage gated K^+ channels close at rest

   Answer: c

• Regular contracting ventricular fibres have a stable resting membrane potential (phase 4), unlike the specialized pacemaker and conducting fibres, which have unstable resting membrane potentials.

• Unlike the skeletal muscle, which has a short action potential, the action potential of the ventricular muscle cell is a long electrical event with a prolonged plateau phase, meaning there can only be one electrical event per mechanical event.

• The single electrical to mechanical event relationship ensures that, unlike the skeletal muscle, the cardiac muscle cell cannot be tetanized.

• Cardiac muscle cells have regions of low electrical resistance between fibres (junctional complexes between fibres including gap junctions) so that action potentials can move from cell to cell as a syncitium.

2. In repolarization:
   a) Ungated K^+ close during repolarization
   b) Voltage gated Na^+ channel open during repolarization
   c) Voltage gated K^+ channel open during repolarization
   d) Calcium channel open during repolarization
   e) Opening of ungated K^+ channel responsible for repolarization

Answer: c

The cardiac muscle cell membrane has channels for K +, Na +, and Ca 2 + ions,

Un-gated K + channels

● These channels are always open and there is always an efflux of K + out of the cardiac muscle cell, as K + equilibrium potential is never reached.

Voltage-dependent (gated) K + channels

● These channels are open at rest.

● They are closed during the plateau phase of the action potential.

● They re-open with repolarization.

Voltage-dependent (gated) Na + channels

● These channels are closed at rest.

● They open quickly and close quickly.

● They are open during depolarization.

Voltage-dependent (gated) Ca 2 + channels

● These channels are closed at rest.

● With depolarization they open and remain open during the plateau phase.

3. During plateau phase:

a) Ungated K^+ channel close during

b) Voltage gated Na^+ channel open

c) Calcium channel open

d) Voltage gated K^+ channel close

e) Both c and d

Answer: e

Cardiac muscle action potential

Phase 0 (depolarization)

● fast Na + channels open.

● the Na + influx into the cell causes the depolarization

Phase 1 (slight repolarization)

● this is thought to be due to special K + rather than Cl − channels.

Phase 2 (plateau)

● the slow voltage-dependent Ca 2 + channels are open, resulting in Ca 2 + influx into the cell.

• the Ca 2 + influx participates in the contractile response and also triggers additional Ca 2 + release from intracellular storage in the sarcoplasmic reticulum.

• voltage-dependent K + channels are closed (only theUn-gated channels are open, so K + conductance is low allowing just the usual efflux of K + but no more).

The Ca 2+ influx balances the K + efflux, which produces the stable plateau phase and delays repolarization.

• The closure of the voltage-dependent K + channels

Ensures that there is no massive efflux of K + , adding to the delay in repolarization .

Phase 3 (repolarization)

• The voltage-dependent Ca 2 + channels close, thereby terminating the Ca 2 + influx.

• Voltage-dependent K + channels re-open, thereby increasing K + efflux and causing repolarization.

4. False statement among following is:

   a) Sympathetic stimulation cause increase intrinsic firing

   b) Pukinje fibres have slowest intrinsic rate

   c) Purkinje fibres have fasted conducting speed

   d) AV node have slowest conducting speed

   e) SA node have fastest conducting velocity

Answer: e

• Sympathetic stimulation increases the slope of the prepotential (phase 4) so that threshold is reached sooner, thus increasing the intrinsic firing rate.

• Parasympathetic stimulation decreases the pre-potential slope so that it takes longer to reach threshold, thus slowing down the intrinsic firing rate.

• SA nodal cells have the fastest intrinsic rate, with AV

Nodal cells being next fastest, and the purkinje fibres have the slowest intrinsic rate.

• However, the purkinje cells are the fastest conducting fibres, whilst the AV node cells are the slowest.

5. Preload is measured by:
   a) Mean aortic pressure
   b) Pulmonary capillary wedge pressure

c) Frank sterling law

d) Pressure in right ventricle

e) Pressure in right atrium

Answer: b

Cardiac muscle mechanics

• Preload is the stretch on the ventricular muscle at the end of diastole. It is measured by the pulmonary capillary edge pressure.

• Left ventricular afterload measured by the mean aortic pressure.

• The Frank–starling relationship is simply the effect of preload on sarcomere length , preload increase ---then increase in length of fibres -----which increases systolic force----which increase cardiac output.

6. Cardiac output is :
   a) 4 l/min
   b) 5 l/min
   c) 6 l/min
   d) 7 l /min
   e) 3 l /min

Answer: b

Cardiac output (CO) in is 5 l/min

7. Most important factor for vascular resistance is:
   a) Radius
   b) Pressure gradient
   c) Flow
   d) Systolic blood pressure
   e) Diastolic blood pressure

Answer: a

• Vessel radius (r) is the chief determinant of vascular resistance. This is expressed in the Poiseuille's relationshion:

$q = p1 - p2/r^4$

Q = fl ow, and p 1 – p 2 = pressure gradient

(i.e. Flow is inversely related to the 4th power of the vessel radius). Thus, if the radius of an arteriole is halved, the resistance increases 16-fold.

Other determinants of vascular resistance include vessel length, blood viscosity, and turbulent flow.

8. MAP=
   a) DBP + SBP
   b) 2/3 DBP+SBP
   c) DBP + 1/3 (pulse pressure)
   d) SBP + 1/3 (pulse pressure)
   e) 1/3DBP + 2/3 SBP

Answer: c

MAP = DBP + ⅓(pulse pressure).

9. False statement among following is:
   a) CO=MAP/SVR
   b) Blood pressure measurement is not good index of acute blood loss
   c) During exercise there is constriction of exercising muscle`s vessel
   d) Cardiac output increase during exercise
   e) During acute blood loss SVR increase and map remain stable

Answer: c

C0=MAP/SVR or

MAP – CO X SVR

In acute blood loss the co falls as a result of volume loss, and the system compensates by vasoconstriction to raise svr and maintain map. Otherwise, map would fall and compromise tissue perfusion. Thus, blood pressure measurement in this situation is not a good index of volume loss. During exercise there is arteriolar dilatation of the exercising muscles (i.e. A reduction in SVR), so the system compensates by increasing the CO to maintain map and avoid compromising tissue perfusion.

10. True statement among following is:

a) If blood pressure decreases there is vasoconstriction in auto regulating tissue

b) Blood pressure determine flow through blood vessel in autoregulating tissue

c) Blood flow is dependant on carotid sinus reflex

d) Autoregulatin of ateriol smooth muscle does not dependent on adrenalin or any nerve

e) In skeletal muscle flow is independent of sympathetic nervous system.

Answer: d

The factors that determine the degree of constriction of the smooth muscle surrounding the arterioles are divided into two categories, namely: intrinsic (or auto) regulation, in which the regulating mechanisms for arteriolar constriction are entirely within the organ itself; and extrinsic regulation, where the mechanisms of arteriolar smooth muscle regulation originate outside of the tissue. Autoregulated systems do not involve any nerves or circulating substances such as adrenaline.

Characteristics of autoregulating tissues

In these tissues BP does not determine flow, and blood flow is independent of BP.

Flow is maintained at a constant level across a wide range of BP . If BP increases, the internal mechanisms constrict the arteriolar smooth muscles and reduce blood flow back to the constant level. If BP falls, the internal mechanisms relax the arterioles to increase the blood flow to the tissues back to the constant level. There are limits to the BP over which such regulation can maintain constant flow, as shown in..

● Blood flow is independent of nervous reflexes such as the carotid sinus reflex.

● Completely autoregulating tissues include the cerebral circulation, coronary circulation, and exercising skeletal muscles .

Characteristics of non-autoregulating (extrinsically regulated) tissues

•Extrinsically regulated tissues include the resting skeletal muscle and the cutaneous circulation.

• The main mechanism for the control of blood flow in all non-autoregulating tissues in the systemic circulation is the sympathetic nervous system, which releases noradrenaline onto the alpha-adrenoceptor under resting conditions.

• The beta2 -receptor is not associated with nervous control but responds mainly to circulating adrenaline causing arteriolar dilatation and contributing to the regulation of blood flow in the resting skeletal muscle.

11. Blood flow through cerebral circulation is directly proportion do
   a) PCO_2
   b) PO_2
   c) CO
   d) Baroreceptor
   e) Both a and d

Answer: a

Characteristics of the cerebral Circulation

• The flow is directly proportional to arterial pCO 2 , the vasodilatory metabolite.

• With hypoventilation, arterial pCO 2 rises and cerebral blood flow increases. During hyperventilation, arterial pCO 2 falls resulting in a fall in cerebral blood flow.

• normal or high pO 2 do not aff ect cerebral blood flow, although a profound reduction in pO 2 will override this mechanism and increase cerebral blood flow regardless of the arterial pCO 2 level.

• Baroreceptor reflexes do not affect cerebral flow.

12. Tachycardia is dangerous because:
   a) Blood flow through left coronary artery mainly during systole
   b) Blood flow through right coronary artery mainly during systole
   c) Blood flow through left coronary artery mainly during diastole

d) During tachycardia systole time decrease more than diastole time so tachycardia is dangerous

e) There is no flow during systole in right coronary artery

Answer: c

● There is severe mechanical compression of the left coronary vessels during systole so that there is little or no flow. Most of the blood flow to the left ventricle is during diastole. This makes severe tachycardia dangerous because of the shortened time interval available for coronary perfusion.

● The right coronary vessels are compressed only to a modest degree during systole so that some flow occurs. However, the greatest flow is during diastole.

● Oxygen extraction from this circuit is complete, a phenomenon that is not observed anywhere else in the body (the venous PO2 is the lowest in the entire cardiovascular system).

● Flow matches metabolism.

13. During cold condition:
   a) Vasoconstriction
   b) Increase velocity of blood flow
   c) Decrease heat exchange and conservation of heat
   d) Increase release of adrenalin
   e) All of above
   Answer: e

14. Characteristic of pulmonary circulation is:
   a) Passive low resistance, low pressure(arterial 15mmhg, venous 5mmhg), high flow, receive entire cardiac output
   b) No sympathetic nerve in pulmonary circulation
   c) Low pO2 in cause vasoconstriction in local alveoli followed by redistribution of blood in alveoli with better blood flow , called hypoxic vasoconstriction

    d) Large change in cardiac output produce very small change in pulmonary circulation

    e) All of above

    Answer: e

15. In pregnancy plasma volume increase by :

    a) 10%

    b) 20%

    c) 30%

    d) 40%

    e) 60%

    Answer: d

Cardiovascular changes in pregnancy:
- Plasma volume is increased by 45–50 %
- Blood volume is increased by 40 %
- Heart rate increases by 10–20 bpm (by 32 weeks)
- Cardiac output is increased by 30–50 % (by 24 weeks)
- Systemic vascular resistance (SVR) is reduced by 20–30 %
- Dilutional decrease in colloid oncotic pressure
- Central venous pressure is unchanged

16. False statement among following is:

    a) Anatomical dead space is part of respiratory system where air present but not exchange with blood, about 150 ml(include conducting airways)

    b) Following normal inspiration dead space has air similar to room air

    c) During inspiration negative intrathorasic pressure goes from -5 to -8 mmhg

    d) In airway partial pressure of oxygen is 160mmhg

    e) None of above

    Answer: d

• The respiratory zone (theoretically in the alveoli) is approximately 2500 ml in volume and should be exchanging with blood. It is considered a constant environment.

• At the end of normal inspiration, the air within the dead space is the same as room air and is generally considered to lack CO_2.

• Following expiration, the air in the dead space has the same composition as that in the respiratory zone.

-During inspiration — the diaphragm — contracts, there is an increase in the negative pressure within the thoracic cavity from –5 mmhg to –8 mmhg.

-The main gases in the atmosphere, N_2, O_2, and CO_2, exert a combined atmospheric pressure of 760 mmhg. Oxygen makes up 21 % of this mixture, or 160 mmhg of the total atmospheric pressure. However, when air is taken into the airway, water vapour is added and this reduces the partial pressure of oxygen from 160 mmhg to 100 mmhg .

17.In adult female tidal volume is :

a) 500
b) 1900
c) 800
d) 1100
e) 4200

Answer: a

Average lung volumes in healthy adults and their measurements

Measurement	Defination	Male	Female
Tidal volume	Volume of air in and out of the lungs During a normal respiratory cycle	500	500

Inspiratory reserve volume	Maximum volume of air that can be inspired Beyond the normal tidal volume	3100	1900
Expiratory reserve volume	Maximum volume of air that can be expired From the resting end-expiratory position	1200	800
Residual volume	Volume of air left in the respiratory system After a maximal expiration; this is the volume Of air that you can	1200	1100

	never expire		

18. In female functional residual capacity is:
   a) 4200
   b) 3100
   c) 2400
   d) 1800
   e) 1100

   Answer: d

Average lung volumes in healthy adults and their measurements

Measurement	Defination	Male	Female
Total lung capacity	Maximum amount of air contained in the lungs after A maximum inspiratory eff ort: TV + IRV + ERV + RV	6000	4200
Vital capacity	Maximum amount of air that can be expired	4800	3100

	after A maximum inspiratory eff ort: TV + IRV + ERV		
Inspiratory capacity	Maximum amount of air that can be inspired After a normal expiration: TV + IRV	3600	2400
Functional residual capacity	Volume of air remaining in the lungs after a Normal tidal volume expiration: ERV + RV	2200	1800

19.False statement among following is:

a) In arterial blood total oxygen content is 19.7 volume %

b) Each haemoglobin molecule carry 1 oxygen molecule

c) On site 1 of hemoglobin molecule oxygen is usually attach in physiological condition

d) On site 2 minimum pO2 require is same as p50

e) On site 4 pO2 require is 100mmhg

Answer: b

Oxygen is carried in two forms in the bloodstream: (i) dissolved in plasma (up to 0.3 volume %); and (ii) carried by haemoglobin (19.4 volume %). 'oxygen content' refers to the concentration of oxygen in the blood expressed in volume % ; in the arterial blood the total oxygen content is 19.7 volume % . Although oxygen is very poorly soluble in plasma, it is the dissolved oxygen that creates PO_2 . PO_2 is the force that keeps oxygen attached to the haemoglobin molecule because haemoglobin does not have suffi cient affinity to bind oxygen in the absence of a PO_2 .

Characteristics of binding sites for O_2 on the Hb molecule (oxyhaemoglobin)

Each haemoglobin molecule contains four iron (Fe^{2+}) ions, each providing an attachment site for an oxygen molecule. Therefore, each haemoglobin molecule can carry a maximum of four oxygen molecules. In the lungs haemoglobin combines with oxygen to form oxyhaemoglobin (HBO_2) with the saturation of the hemoglobin molecule dependent on the amount of oxygen in the alveolar air. The four binding sites on the Hb molecule are specific and ranked from 1 to 4 depending on the strength of their affinity (the higher the affinity of the binding site, the smaller the PO_2 required for binding).

• Site 1 — oxygen is usually attached to this site under physiological conditions.

• Site 2 — minimum PO_2 for oxygen to bind to this site is 26 mmhg, which is also the p 50 for oxygen binding to Hb (PO_2 required for 50 % of the Hb to be saturated with oxygen).

• Site 3 — minimum pO_2 for oxygen binding to this site is 40 mmhg, which is also the pO_2 of systemic venous blood. Venous blood is thus 75 % saturated under resting conditions, meaning only one molecule of oxygen is extracted from the Hb molecule in the tissues.

• Site 4 has the least affinity for oxygen and therefore needs the greatest pO_2 to keep oxygen attached to the haemoglobin molecule. The pO_2 for binding to this site is 100 mmhg and thus Hb is 97 % saturated when leaving the lungs.

20. Which factor does not shift oxygen dissociation curve to right
    a) Increase CO2
    b) Decrease Ph
    c) Increase temperature
    d) Decrease DPG
    e) Increase DPG
       Answer: d

Haemoglobin is most attracted to oxygen when three of the four binding sites are bound to oxygen.

Factors affecting the oxygen–haemoglobin Dissociation curve

If the curve is shifted to the right, the p 50 moves to the right, meaning that a higher PO2 is required to keep oxygen attached to the haemoglobin molecule. In Other words, there is a loss of affinity and systemic tissues will find it easier to get oxygen from the haemoglobin molecule.

• *Temperature* — increasing the temperature
• *Carbon dioxide and acidity (ph)* — CO2 decreases the Ph and this causes oxyhaemoglobin to dissociate and release O2 . A very small decrease in the ph results in a large decrease in the percentage saturation of the haemoglobin with O2 . The shift of the dissociation curve to the right when the ph is low even with a relatively high PO 2 is called the *bohr effect* .
• *2,3-diphosphoglycerate (DPG)* — the primary mammalian organic phosphate binds to haemoglobin and rearranges the haemoglobin molecule in a way that decreases its affinity for oxygen, and shifts the curve to the right. If the curve is shifted to the left, there is a gain in haemoglobin affinity for oxygen.

Therefore, it is easier to load haemoglobin with oxygen in the lungs but more difficult for the tissues to extract oxygen.

Factors that shift the oxygen dissociation curve to the left include:

• Reduced temperature, reduced PCO_2 , reduced 2,3-DPG, reduced H + (or raised ph), fetal haemoglobin, and myoglobin .

• Carbon monoxide — this shifts the curve to the left because it increases haemoglobin affinity for oxygen, but also shifts it downwards because it reduces saturation of the haemoglobin.

In simple anaemia, the oxygen saturation is normal but the overall oxygen content of the blood (oxygen-carrying capacity) is reduced because of the reduced Hb concentration. With polycythaemia there is more oxygen contained per unit volume. In both anaemia and polycythaemia, the curve does not shift.

21.95 % of carbondioxide is transported as:

a) Dissolved CO2
b) Carbamino compund
c) Bicarbonate
d) None of above
e) B and c

Answer: c

Carbon dioxide transport

Co2 is carried in three forms:

1. Dissolved carbon dioxide

2. Carbamino (protein) compounds (HbCo 2)

3. Bicarbonate (HCO3 –) (most CO2 is carried as plasma HCO3 –).

• within the capillaries of systemic tissues, the CO 2

Produced is picked up by the RBC, where the reaction

Co 2 + H 2 O ↔H+ + HCO 3 – takes place, catalysed by the enzyme carbonic anhydrase. The H + is buffered by the hb molecule whilst the HCO 3 – is transported back out of the cell into the plasma, where it is transported. Chloride ions (cl –) move into the RBC to maintain electrical neutrality. Around 95 % of the CO 2 generated in the tissues is carried as bicarbonate in this way.

• When the RBC reach the lungs these reactions are reversed, with HCO3 – entering the RBC to combine with H + to form water and co 2. Chloride ions exit the RBC to maintain electrical neutrality(chloride shift). The CO 2 is released to the air of the alveoli.

• Approximately 5 % of the CO 2 generated in the tissues dissolves directly in the plasma (but if all the CO2 generated were carried in the plasma, the ph of the blood would drop from 7.4 to a fatal 4.5).

22. Which of following stimulate central chemoreceptor and cross blood brain barrier:
   a) Co2
   b) O2
   c) H+ ions
   d) OH-
   e) HCO-
   Answer: a

Central chemoreceptor: CO2 & H+ act on this but H+ ion cannot cross blood brain barrier so CO2 act as main factor peripheral chemoreceptor: respond to CO2 , O2

23. Changes in respiratory system in pregnancy:
   a) Oxygen demand increases
   b) Functional residual capacity reduced
   c) Minute ventilation increases
   d) Respiratory rate increases
   e) All of above
   Answer: e

Pregnancy-specific changes in the respiratory system

• Oxygen demand is increased.
• Functional residual capacity (FRC) is reduced.
• Oxygen desaturation is more common.
• Minute ventilation is increased.

- Respiratory rate is increased.
- Mild respiratory alkalosis.

24. Kidney secrets and containt:
    a) Erythropiotin
    b) Renin
    c) 1,25 hydroxyl cholecalciferol
    d) 1 million nephron
    e) All of above
    Answer: e

25. ADH act on:
    a) Proximal convoluted tubule
    b) Distal convoluted tubule
    c) Loop of henle
    d) Collecting duct
    e) Glomerular tuft
    Answer: d

26. Kidney receive % of cardiac output:
    a) 10-15%
    b) 15-20%
    c) 20-25%
    d) 35-45%
    e) 45-55%
    Answer: c

- The kidneys normally receive 20–25 % of the total cardiac output.
- The glomerular filtration rate (GFR) is the amount of filtrate produced from the blood per unit time. The gfr in non-pregnant individuals is 90–120 ml/min/1.73 m 2 of surface area and about 180 l of filtrate is produced each day.
- The filtration fraction is the proportion of renal plasma flow that gets filtered through the glomerulus, and in normal individuals it is approximately 20 % .
- The glomerular filtrate normally contains no blood cells or platelets, and virtually no protein.

27. Renin is produced by:
    a) Afferent arteriol
    b) Efferent arteriol
    c) Juxtaglomerular apparatus
    d) Collecting duct
    e) Bowmen`s capsule
       Answer: c

The renin-angiotensin-aldosterone system: renin is released by cells of the juxtaglomerular apparatus (JGA) in response to reduced sodium delivery to this part of the nephron or a reduction in renal perfusion pressure.

28. Which of following not occur in pregnancy
    a) Kidney size increase by 1.5 cm
    b) Right ureter dilated more than left ureter
    c) 30% pregnant women develop asymptomatic bacteriuria
    d) There is decrease in risk of urinary tract infection in pregnancy
    e) Sigmoid colon is responsible for dextrorotation of uterus
       Answer: d

Renal physiology in pregnancy
The kidneys increase in size by up to 1.5 cm in bipolar diameter. The collecting system and ureters dilate.
Hydronephrosis is present in up to 90 % of women by the third trimester and is typically more prominent on the right side because of the dextro-rotation of the uterus (which is believed to be at least in part due to the location of the sigmoid colon on the left side) and/or the kinking of the right ureter as it crosses vascular structures.dilatation of the ureters may persist for several weeks postpartum.
The dilated collecting system can hold 200 to 300 ml of urine, which can act as a reservoir for bacteria. There may be intermittent vesico-ureteral reflux during pregnancy. These factors lead to an increased risk of ascending infection. If untreated, 30 % of pregnant women with asymptomatic

bacteriuria will develop pyelonephritis with an increased risk of miscarriage or preterm delivery.

29. Which of following is pathological for pregnancy:
    a) Cardiac output is increased by 30 to 50%
    b) Heart rate increase by 15 beats per minute
    c) 30 to 50 % increase in plasma volume
    d) Reduction in both systolic and diastolic blood pressure
    e) Increase response to angiotensin
       Answer: e

1. *Increase in cardiac output*
During normal pregnancy, the cardiac output (CO) rises by 30 % −50 % as a result of increases both in stroke volume (SV) and heart rate (HR). One half of this increase occurs by 8 weeks of gestation. Stroke volume increases early in pregnancy due to the combination of an increased preload (increased blood volume) and a reduction in afterload, which results from systemic vasodilatation. The baseline heart rate rises by 15 to 20 beats per minute and is the major contributing factor to the increased cardiac output in late pregnancy.

2. *Blood volume expansion*
Salt and water retention leads to a 30 % −50 % expansion in plasma volume at term above non-pregnant levels. The high renin levels observed during pregnancy suggest that the increased plasma volume is a response to the relative under-filling that results from the profound systemic vasodilatation.

3. *Reductions in blood pressure and systemic Vascular resistance (SVR)*
As cardiac output increases there is a marked decrease in systemic vascular resistance, resulting in a modest reduction in arterial blood pressure. The precise mechanism behind the vasodilatation is not fully understood. Contributing factors are likely to include a reduced responsiveness to the vasoconstrictive actions of angiotensin II, increased endothelial prostacyclin, and increased production of nitric oxide .

30. False statement among following is:
    a) Effective renal plasma flow increase by 80% in first and second trimester. And fall to 60% of non pregnant state near term
    b) GFR increase by 50% of normal state
    c) Glomerular autoregulation set at high point in pregnancy
    d) Total no of nephron increase in pregnancy
    e) Reduction in filtration fraction in pregnancy
    Answer: d

GFR increases markedly during pregnancy, and peaks at about 50 % above non-pregnant levels by 16 weeks gestation.
-There is no change in the total number of nephrons.
-Reduction in the 'filtration fraction' during pregnancy.

31. GFR is measured by:
    a) Serum creatinine
    b) Serum uric acid
    c) Serum sodium
    d) Urinary creatinine
    e) Urinary billirubin
    Answer: a

Estimation of GFR during pregnancy
Due to changes in ERPF and GFR, CRCL increases (i.e. Serum creatinine concentration drops) by 25 % in the first 4 weeks and by 40 % –50 % by the end of the first trimester of pregnancy. CRCL decreases by up to 20 % in the third trimester and may increase sliGHtly postpartum, returning to pre-pregnancy levels within 3 months of delivery.
CRCL approximates renal function but is not an exact Measure of GFR.
● These changes in GFR during pregnancy should alert clinicians that a serum creatinine in the normal range during pregnancy is likely to be abnormal and may indicate renal pathology.

32. ADH act on :
   a) Collecting duct
   b) Distal convoluted tubule
   c) Direct vasoconstrictor effect
   d) Aquaporins channel
   e) All of above
   Answer: e

Antidiuretic hormone (ADH) release from thePosterior pituitary. ADH acts on the distal convoluted tubules and collecting duct epithelial cells to stimulate water reabsorption by the insertion of preformed water channels (aquaporins) into the apical membranes. It also has moderate direct vasoconstrictive effects.

33. False statement among following :
   a) Aldosterone secreted from adrena cortex
   b) Aldosterone act on distal collecting tubule and collecting duct and absorb Na+ ions
   c) Aldosterone and angiotensin ii stimulate thirst and salt craving
   d) Hypovolemia leads to decrease specific gravity
   e) Hypervolumia leads to increase in specific gravity
   Answer: d

Increasing aldosterone secretion from the adrenal cortex. Aldosterone acts on distal convoluted tubules and the cortical collecting ducts in the kidneys, enhancing sodium and water reabsorption in exchange for potassium. Aldosterone and angiotensin ii stimulate thirst and salt craving centrally. Taken together, these effects increase BP.
angiotensin II also causes efferent renal arteriolar vasoconstriction to maintain glomerular filtration pressure (and GFR) during reduced renal perfusion. Hypovolaemia leads to production of low volumes of urine that are highly concentrated (> 350 mosm/kg with specifi c gravity > 1.020) but low in sodium (<10 meq/l; fractional excretion of sodium, fena <1 %). In contrast, if hypovolaemia continues and acute tubular injury

supervenes, the effects of the raas are diminished and a salt-losing state with defective concentrating ability supervenes. Established acute tubular injury is, therefore characterized by variable volumes of dilute urine (<350 mosm/kg with specific gravity ≤ 1.010) that are high in sodium (> 40 meq/l; fena > 2%).

34. Which of following is pathological change in pregnancy:
    a) Plasma osmolality drop by 10 mosm/kg during pregnancy
    b) Upward resetting of osmostat
    c) Serum sodium drop by 5 meq/l
    d) PCO2 drop by 10mmhg
    e) Respirator alkosis in pregnancy
       Answer: b

Plasma osmolality drops by about 10 mosm/kg during pregnancy. In a normal and healthy non-pregnant individual, this drop in osmolality should lead to inhibition of ADH and diuresis. However, the osmotic threshold for ADH release also drops during early pregnancy — the so-called 'downward' resetting of the osmostat. The drop in osmotic threshold correlates closely with levels of beta-hcg, which is thought to act indirectly by inducing the release of the hormone relaxin.

-serum sodium drops by about 5 meq/l during pregnancy. The hyponatraemia is not compensated for due to the 'downward' resetting of the osmostat and this resetting of the osmostat means that the lower serum sodium concentration will be maintained at this level despite marked daily variations in sodium or water intake.

The clinical sequelae of the changes in osmolality andSerum sodium is that polyuria is uncommon, as mostWomen can compensate for the higher catabolism ofADH by its increased production. However, polyuria *Can* occur in women with overt or subclinical centralor nephrogenic diabetes insipidus in whom secretory reserve of ADH or renal responsiveness to ADH isImpaired (exacerbated by the rise in GFR seen inPregnancy).

Acid-base balance and potassium

The daily production of metabolic acids is increased in Pregnancy due to an increase in basal metabolic rate, fetal metabolic load, and an increase in daily protein intake.

Pregnancy is characterized by relative alkalaemia: a mean arterial ph of 7.44 (7.40 non-pregnant state) due to hyperventilation induced by progesterone on the respiratory centre and increased respiratory effort in response to the uterus splinting the diaphragm.

There is an overall drop in arterial PCO 2 of about10 mmhg (1.3 kpa) and a compensatory renal loss ofBicarbonate, which partially compensates the ph but results in a lower serum bicarbonate of around 18–22 Mmol/l during pregnancy. In acid-base terms, this could be described as a **metabolic acidosis with respiratory alkalaemia**.

35. In acidosis:

a) Decrease in H+ in extracellular compartment
b) Increase in K+ ion in extracellular compartment
c) PCO2 decrease
d) Decrease in H+ ion in extracellular compartment
e) None of above
Answer: b

Potassium excretion is generally linked to acid-base balance. Acidosis is usually associated with hyperkalaemia and alkalosis with hypokalaemia. Acidosis is characterized by high concentrations of H + in the extracellular fluid compartment. Over time, H + flows into the intracellular compartment. To maintain electrical neutrality, K+ ions are forced out of the intracellular compartment into the extracellular space, creating a state of hyperkalaemia. In alkalosis, the reduced H + concentration in the extracellular fluid compartment is compensated for by an efflux of intracellular H + into the extracellular space. K + flows into the cells to maintain electrical neutrality, creating a
Hypokalaemic state.

36. In pregnancy because of k+ changes :

a) Sickle cell disease is more dangerous
b) conn`s syndrome and barter`s syndrome are dangerous

c) Increase in sensitivity to kaliuric drugs

d) Increase level of progesterone have mineralocorticoid like action

e) All of above

Answer: a

Potassium excretion is reduced during pregnancy despite high aldosterone levels and relatively alkaline urine. The mechanism is not completely understood but it is likely to be related to the elevated levels of progesterone exerting anti-mineralocorticoid effects, probably through the inhibition of active potassium excretion in the distal tubule and collecting ducts. As a result there is net potassium retention, which, like sodium, is distributed throughout fetal and maternal tissues without causing hyperkalaemia.

Clinically, changes in potassium homeostasis result in a relative resistance to kaliuretic drugs (e.g. Mineralocorticoids) and protection against potassium-losing diseases in pregnancy (e.g. Conn's or Bartter's syndromes). Diseases that impair excretion of potassium, such as sickle cell disease, could become more dangerous in pregnancy.

37. In pregnancy:

a) Increase in calcium excretion

b) Increase in calcitriol level

c) Magnesium and citrate level increase

d) Hypocalcaemia is rare

e) All of above

Answer: e

Increased filtered load of calcium to the tubules, resulting in increased calcium excretion.

Elevated levels of calcitriol (1,25-dihydroxy-vitamin D3) suppress the counter-regulatory hormone, parathyroid hormone (PTH), but hypocalcaemia remains rare because calcitriol also stimulates calcium absorption from the gut.

Renal stone formation is rare as urinary 'solubilizing Agents', such as magnesium and citrate, are also high in pregnancy and maintain calcium in solution.

38. Which of following is pathological in pregnancy:

a) Glycosuria
b) Increase in clearance of uric acid
c) Proteinuria more than 300 mg in 24 hour sample
d) Serum level more than 20 mg /dl
e) None of above
   Answer: c

-Glycosuria can be common in pregnancy and is not diagnostic of gestational diabetes.

-Reduced tubular reabsorption of uric acid (i.e. Increased uric acid clearance) causes lowered serum levels of urate during early pregnancy. Often, serum uric acid levels are reduced by about 25 % .

-Proteins are not normally filtered by the glomerulus because of their large size and charge. Increased GFR and glomerular permeability increase filtered levels of proteins during pregnancy. Consequently, both urinary total protein and albumin excretion increase. This is most apparent after about 20 weeks of gestation.

-Proteinuria exceeds 300 mg per 24 hours - abnormal

-In practice the protein to creatinine ratio on a spot sample of urine is more convenient, saves time, and minimizes errors in sample collection.

-The diagnosis of proteinuria can be made with a urine dipstick, but will also require a further method of quantification, such as the urine protein to creatinine ratio on a spot sample or a 24-hour collection.

-Proteinuria can be nephrotic (≥ 3 g per 24 h) or subnephrotic (<3 g per 24 h) in range. Quantification is essential as management of nephrotic-range proteinuria differs from that for sub-nephrotic proteinuria.

Nephrotic syndrome in pregnancy

This is characterized by the triad of significant proteinuria, hypoalbuminaemia, and oedema. The proteinuria is often greater than 3 g per day and can be due to a primary glomerular disease (e.g. Minimal change nephropathy), a systemic disease such as diabetes, or a manifestation of pre-eclampsia.

There is loss of anticoagulant proteins in the urine and the risk of venous thromboembolic disease is high, especially if the albumin level falls below 20 mg/dl. Prophylactic anticoagulation should be considered.

39. Microscopic haematuria in pregnancy due to:
   a) Urinary tract infection
   b) Glomerulonephritis
   c) Henoch-schoenlein purpura
   d) IgA nephropathy
   e) All of above
      Answer: e

Macroscopic (visible) haematuria ensues with ≥ 5 ml of blood/l. Leakage of blood from glomeruli is often accompanied by leakage of protein (blood contains approximately 60 g/l of total protein, of which 40 g/l is albumin) so haematuria accompanied by significant proteinuria usually indicates a glomerular source for the haematuria. Lower quantities of haematuria are not usually visible to the naked eye (microscopic haematuria).

Microscopic haematuria (non-visible) in pregnancy could be due to a urinary tract infection, glomerulonephritis, or pre-eclampsia. Macroscopic haematuria is more likely to be due to contamination from vaginal bleeding or a urinary tract infection, but can be seen in some glomerular diseases such as iga nephropathy or henoch-schoenlein purpura (HSP).

40. Site of hematopiosis in embryo is:
   a) Yolk sac
   b) liver
   c) Bone marrow
   d) Vertebrae
   e) Skull
      Answer: a

Blood consists of 55 % plasma and 45 % cellular components (99 % of which are red blood cells and 1 white blood cells and platelets).
The site of haematopoiesis varies with age:
In the early embryo it is first seen in the yolk sac.

In infants it occurs in fetal liver and throuGHout the Bone marrow (BM).

By adulthood it occurs in the BM of the central skeleton (vertebrae, ribs, sternum, skull, sacrum, pelvis) and in proximal ends of long bones (humerus and femur).

The haematopoietic stem cell (HSC) is the earliest cell that can be identified in BM. It is pluripotent: capable of self-renewal and of differentiating into all cell lineages including red cells, white cells, and platelets.

41. Which of following is not physiological change in pregnancy:
    a) Increase in red cell mass by 30%
    b) Increase in plasma volume by 30%
    c) Decrease in MCV
    d) Increase in coagulation factors
    e) Decrease in platelet count by 10%

    Answer: c

Physiological changes in pregnancy
Increased red cell mass by up to 30 % .
Increased plasma volume by up to 60 % .
Net increase in blood volume of up to 50 % .
Decreased haemoglobin concentration and haematocrit.
Increased MCV.
Decreased platelet count by up to 10 % .
Increased level of coagulation factors

42. Which of following is wrong about RBC:
    a) Biconcave disc with no nucleus
    b) Do not contain DNA, RNA and mitochondria
    c) Average life span 120 days
    d) Erythropoietin is produced by interstitial cells of kidney
    e) Erythropoietin use for treatment of chronic anemia in renal failure

    Answer: d

Red blood cells (RBC)

- They are large (about 6–8 μm) biconcave discs with no nucleus.
- There are about 4.5–5.8 million RBC/ μ l (with gender and racial variation).
- Their main role is to transport oxygen from the lungs to the body tissues, but they also transfer carbon dioxide from the tissues to be exhaled by the lungs.
- They do not contain DNA, RNA, or mitochondria and Produce energy (ATP) from glycolysis throuGH the reducing power of NADH and NADPH.
- the average life span of each RBC is 120 days.
- production is regulated by the growth factor erythropoietin (EPO).

Epo
- EPO is produced in peritubular cells of the kidney.
- It is released at low O2 tension (hypoxia, anaemia).
- It reacts with epo receptors on rbc precursors to Increase production ≥ 6-fold.
- Recombinant EPO is now available for the treatment of anaemia due to renal failure and for Jehovah's witness patients who decline transfusion of allogenic blood components on religious grounds.

43. Which of following is correct about haemoglobin
   a) It is pentameric molecule
   b) Shift of HbA to HbF start at 6 month of age
   c) 1 gram of haemoglobin combine with 1.34 ml of o2
   d) Absorption of iron is mainly in ferrous form
   e) Normal store of vitamin B 12 is 2 to 4 mg which remain for 2 to 4 days

   Answer: c

Haemoglobin
- This is a tetrameric molecule containing four haem groups and four globin chains. Haem is a ferrous iron molecule in a porphyrin ring structure and globin is a polypeptide chain containing two alpha chains and two non alpha chains.
- Adult Hb (HbA) is made up of two alpha and two beta globin chains.

• Fetal Hb (HbF) is made up of two alpha and two beta chains; the switch from HbF to HbA starts at birth and is complete by about 6 months.

• It is important for oxygen transport from the lungs, where there is a high partial pressure of oxygen (pO_2), to the tissues, with a low pO_2. On average, 1 g of Hb combines with 1.34 ml of O_2.

Haematinics: dietary substances essential for the production of RBC and Hb

iron

combines with Protoporphyrin ring to form haem (there are four haem groups to each tetramer of Hb).

• Found in food as ferric hydroxide, ferric protein complexes, and haem protein complexes, with red meat being the best source available. Normal daily intake from a western diet is 10–15 mg but only 1–2 mg (5–10 %) is absorbed daily.

• Absorption occurs in the duodenum and jejunum, mainly in the ferric form, enhanced by acid and reducing agents, E.g. Ascorbic acid.

• Transported in plasma combined with transferrin and Stored as ferritin.

• Increased iron is required in pregnancy and lactation.

Vitamin B 12

• Produced only by micro-organisms and found mainly in animal produce.

• Absorption occurs through the ileum in combination with intrinsic factor (IF), which is produced by gastric parietal cells.

• Minimum daily requirement of 1–2 µg; normal body Stores of 2–3 mg last 2–4 years.

44. Daily requirement of folic acid is:
    a) 100 to 200 mcg
    b) 200 to 400 mcg
    c) 400 to 600 mcg
    d) 10 to 20 mg
    e) 20 to 40 mg
        Answer: a

Natural folates in the polyglutamate form occur in most foods but especially liver, vegetables, and yeasts; however,they are easily destroyed by cooking.

• Absorption is through the duodenum and jejunum.

• Normal daily dietary intake of 600–1000 μ g; daily requirement of 100–200 μ g and body stores of 10–12 mg last for up to 4 months.

45. Which of following is incorrect

   a) Size of neutrophil is 10 to 12 micrometer
   b) Eoisinophil has 3 lobed nuclei and coarse red granular cytoplasm
   c) Basophil involved in immediate hypersensitivity reaction
   d) Monocyte produce antibodies
   e) Life span of platelet is 7 to 10 days

   Answer: d

White blood cells (WBC)

Average life span of a few hours to a few days.

WBC include both granulocytes and agranular leukocytes.

Granulocytes (or polymorphs)

These have large, characteristic granules in their cytoplasm that can be seen under a light microscope. They are much smaller than the RBC, averaging about 1/700 of a RBC.

There are three types of granulocytes: neutrophils, eosinophils, and basophils.

(a) Neutrophils

Average size is 10–12 μm in diameter.

There is a dense nucleus made of two to five lobes connected by thin strands of chromatin, and the cytoplasm has very fine, pale lilac granules.

Attracted to sites of infection/inflammation by chemotaxis, where they phagocytose and kill bacteria.

Neutrophil leukocytosis or an increase in neutrophil numbers occurs mostly in infection but also in pregnancy, exercise, stress, steroid treatment, and myeloproliferative disorders.

• *Neutropenia* or a decrease in numbers occurs with bone marrow failure syndromes, drugs, viral infections, and autoimmune disorders. Severe neutropenia ($<1.0 \times 10^9$ /l) can lead to life-threatening infections.

(b) Eosinophils

• Nuclei have up to three lobes and the cytoplasm contains coarser pink/red granules.

• Play an important role in specific defence against parasites and in response to allergic reactions.

(c) Basophils

• Have bi-lobed nuclei and contain large, dark-purple Cytoplasmic granules.

• Involved in immediate hypersensitivity reactions (asthma, anaphylaxis) and in defence against allergens and parasites.

Agranulocytes

Agranulocytes do not contain visible granules. They include lymphocytes and monocytes:

• *Lymphocytes* produce antibodies including T cells, B cells, and NK cells.

• *Monocytes* are essential for active phagocytosis of bacteria.

Platelets

• Small (2–4 μ m), non-nucleated cells with a complex infrastructure including numerous cytoplasmic granules.

• Production occurs in bm by fragmentation of the cytoplasm of their precursor, the megakaryocyte (very large, multi-nucleated cells found only in bm).

• Production is regulated by the growth factor thrombopoietin, which is produced mainly in the liver.

• Platelets play a vital role in the primary haemostatic Process.

• normal life span is 7–10 days.

46. In iron deficiency anemia:
   a) Microcytic hypochromic anemia
   b) Valin substituted by glutamic acid on beta chain at 6 th position
   c) Mutation in alpha or beta globulin chain
   d) Vitamin b12 or folic acid deficiency
   e) Associated with autoimmune disorder

Answer: a

Anaemia in pregnancy can be:

- Dilutional anaemia (Hb rarely <10.0 g/dl)
- Microcytic anaemia (low MCV) in iron deficiency anaemia, haemoglobinopathies
- Macrocytic anaemia (high MCV) in folate deficiency(common), vitamin B 12 deficiency (rare).
- Anaemia due to other chronic underlying disorder.

Microcytic anaemia

(a) Iron deficiency anaemia

Blood film shows microcytic, hypochromic red cells.

Management

Treat underlying cause.

Oral iron (ferrous sulphate; 67 mg elemental iron per 200 mg tablet) for up to 6 months to correct anaemia and replenish stores:

Expected Hb rise of about 2 g/dl every 3 weeks.

Constipation is main side effect managed by reducing dose or using preparation with a lower iron content, e.g. Ferrous gluconate (37 mg iron/300 mg tablet).

Parenteral iron is available but may cause allergic

Reactions or anaphylaxis.

Blood transfusion rarely indicated.

(b) Haemoglobinopathies

- Sickle cell disease: single amino acid substitution occurs on beta chain (valine substituted for glutamic acid at position 6).
- Thalassaemias: mutations in one or more of the alpha or beta globin genes cause a reduction in the amount of HbA produced. Pernicious anaemia (PA) is associated with other autoimmune disorders (e.g. Myxoedema, addison's disease) and an increased risk of gastric carcinoma.

47.Recommended dose of folic acid for prophylaxis is:
   a) 400mcg
   b) 5mg
   c) 1000mcg
   d) 200mcg
   e) 100 mcg

Answer: a

Prophylaxis in pregnancy: deficiency in pregnancy is associated with neural tube defects in the fetus, although there is no clear correlation between maternal folate levels and the occurrence of defects. However, folic acid supplement in early pregnancy (400 µ g daily from conception) reduces the incidence of spina bifida, anencephaly, and cleft lip and palate. The higher daily dose of 5 mg is recommended for women on antiepileptic drugs as these agents have antifolate properties.

Table 3.5 iron defi ciency anaemia
Iron studies   (normal values)
Serum iron: ↓(10–30 µmol/l)
Total iron binding capacity: ↑ (50–70 µmol/l)
Transferrin saturation: ↓ (> 16 %)
Serum ferritin level: ↓ (12–150 µg/l)

48. Macrocytosisi is caused by:
   a) Reticulocytosis
   b) Vitamin B12 deficiency
   c) Alcoholic liver disease
   d) Hypothyroidism
   e) All of above
      Answer: e

Macrocytosis can be caused by any of the following:
- Reticulocytosis (acute bleeding)
- Vitamin B 12 or folate deficiency
- Alcoholic liver disease
- Hypothyroidism
- Myelodysplasia.

49. Vitamin B12 deficiency is caused by:
   a) Vegetarian
   b) Pernicious anemia
   c) Blind loop syndrome
   d) Malabsorption
   e) All of above
      Answer: e

(a) Vitamin B 12 deficiency
May be caused by:
Malabsorption
Dietary lack (vegans)
Pernicious anaemia: antibodies against intrinsic factor
Blind-loop syndrome.
Presents with macrocytic, megaloblastic anaemia but severe deficiency may cause neurological complications such as subacute combined degeneration of the cord.

- Pernicious anaemia (PA) is associated with other autoimmune disorders (e.g. Myxoedema, addison's disease) and an increased risk of gastric carcinoma.
- Investigations:
- Radioactive vitamin B 12 absorption + /– if (schilling test)
- Serum gastric parietal and intrinsic factor antibodies
- Endoscopy: gastric/duodenal biopsy
- Treat underlying cause; replace stores with parenteral B 12 (hydroxycobalamin):
- Initial/loading dose of 1 mg every 3–4 days for up to 6doses
- Maintenance dose of 1 mg every 3 months.

(b) Folic acid deficiency
- May be caused by:
Inadequate dietary intake
Malabsorption: coeliac disease, tropical sprue
Increased requirements: pregnancy, haemolysis
Drugs, e.g. Anticonvulsantexcess alcohol intake.
- Investigations:
Serum folate levels ; serum B 12 levels
Antigliadin and Endomysial antibodies
Tests for malabsorption, e.g. Duodenal biopsy
- Treat underlying cause and replace stores with oral folic acid (5 mg daily).
- Prior to replacement with folic acid, B 12 defi ciency must be excluded and treated to prevent development or exacerbation of neurological complications.
- Prophylaxis in pregnancy: deficiency in pregnancy is associated with neural tube defects in the fetus, although there is no clear correlation between maternal folate levels and the occurrence of defects. However, folic acid supplement in early

pregnancy (400 μ g daily from conception) reduces the incidence of spinabifida, anencephaly, and cleft lip and palate. The higher daily dose of 5 mg is recommended for women on antiepileptic drugs as these agents have antifolate properties.

50. Causes of disseminated intravascular coagulation in pregnancy:
    a) Placental abruption
    b) Eclampsia
    c) Amniotic fluid embolism
    d) Intrauterine infection
    e) All of above
       Answer: e

DICin pregnancy it is associated with:
Massive haemorrhage
Septic miscarriage and intra-uterine infection
Pre-eclampsia/eclampsia
Abruptio placentae
Retained dead fetus
Amniotic fluid embolism
Hydatidiform mole.

51. In DIC
    a) Increase platelet count
    b) Decrease PT,APTT,TT
    c) Decrease fibriogen
    d) Increase fibrinogen degradation product
    e) Decrease neutrophil count
       Answer: d

Diagnosis is confirmed by haematological investigations:
Decrease platelet count
Increase PT, APTT
Increase fibrinogen
Increase fibrinogen degradation products .
Increase cross-linked fibrin degradation products (d-dimers)

Treatment includes the replacement of blood products (platelets, FFP, cryoprecipitate) and urgent treatment of the underlying condition.

52. Features of hellp syndrome is:
    a) Haemolysis
    b) Elevated liver enzyme
    c) Low platelet count
    d) Only b and c
    e) A , b and c
       Answer: e

HELLP syndrome
Microangiopathic haemolysis (H), elevated liver enzymes (EL), low platelets (LP).
• Occurs in severe pre-eclampsia.
• Laboratory findings as in DIC.
• Mainstay of treatment is delivery, although corticosteroids have been used.

53. Which of following change is not responsible for thromboembolism in pregnancy:
    a) Decrease fibrinogen
    b) Increase vitamin K dependent factors
    c) Increase factor VII
    d) Hyperhomocysteinaemia
    e) Factor V leiden mutation
       Answer: a

Pregnancy is a hypercoagulable state and pulmonary embolism (PE) remains a major cause of maternal death. The following physiological changes in coagulation factors occur in pregnancy:
• Increase levels of vitamin K-dependent factors (II, VII, IX, and X)
• Increase factor VIII and Von Willebrand factor levels
• Increase fibrinogen levels
• Increase in levels of coagulation inhibitors (protein C, antithrombin III).

Other risk factors for thromoboembolism in pregnancy
Include:

• Previous thrombotic history

• Obesity

• Caesarean section or other recent major surgery

• Inherited pro-thrombotic states or familial thrombophilia due to deficiency of coagulation inhibitors (protein C, protein S, antithrombin III), factor V leiden gene mutation, or activated protein C resistance and hyperhomocysteinaemia.

-Thrombocytopenia in pregnancy

• *Incidental* or *Gestational* thrombocytopenia accounts for 75 % of cases of mild to moderately low platelet counts (70–150 × 10 9 /l). Characteristically, there is no previous history and no clinical effect on the baby. *Autoimmune thrombocytopenia* is caused by an antiplatelet autoantibody (IgG), which may cross the placenta and destroy fetal platelets.

54. Not transmission transmissible infection:

   a) Hepatitis B

   b) Streptoccoci

   c) HIV

   d) CMV

   e) Malaria

   Answer: b

Rhesus blood group

• discovered by Karl Landsteiner and A.S. Wiener in 1941. The most significant rhesus antigen is the RH D antigen because it is the most immunogenic of the five main rhesus antigens.

Transfusion transmissible infections

• viruses: hepatitis A, B, and C; HIV-i and ii; CMV

• bacteria: *treponema pallidum* (syphilis); brucella; salmonella

• parasites: malaria; toxoplasma; microfilaria

• prion protein: Creutzfeldt–Jakob disease (CJD) and new variant CJD (NVCJD)

55. Intramascular anti-D is given at:

   a) 28

   b) 34

   c) Within 72 hour of delivery

d) A, b ,c
e) A and b only

Answer: d

56. Fetal cells in maternal blood using:
   a) Kleihauer- Betke test
   b) Shirodkar test
   c) Budha`s test
   d) Apt test
   e) Londersloot test

   Answer: a

Haemolytic disease of the newborn (HDN)

• This is transplacental passage of maternal red cell IgG antibodies resulting in haemolysis of fetal RBC.

• the *most frequent* cause is ABO incompatibility, e.g. Anti- A produced by a group O mother carrying a group A fetus. The disease is usually mild because ABO antibodies are IgM, which are large molecules and less likely to cross the placenta. Furthermore, maternal antibodies are partially neutralized by A and B antigens on other cells, plasma, and tissue fluids.

• the *most important* cause of HDN is anti-D, although otherRH antibodies (particularly anti-C and anti-Kell) are also implicated.

• Clinical features include anaemia, neonatal jaundice (resulting in kernicterus in severe cases), hydrops fetalis, and intra-uterine death (IUD).

• Treatment includes phototherapy in mild cases and red cell exchange transfusions for severe jaundice.

• Prophylactic anti-D IgG is given to rh (D)-negative women within 72 hours of a potentially sensitizing event. The dose is adjusted according to the number of fetal cells detected in maternal circulation using the Kleihauer- Betke test.

• In the UK routine antenatal prophylaxis against rhesus disease is recommended. Intramuscular anti-d 1250 IU is routinely administered to all pregnant RH D-negative women at 28 weeks and 34 weeks gestation.

SBA MRCOG PART 1

57.Immunoglobulin which crosses placenta is:
   a) IgG
   b) IgM
   c) IgD
   d) IgE
   e) IgA
      Answer: a

Antibodies can be divided into five classes, or nine subclasses,corresponding to the nine isotypes.
The immunoglobulin G (IgG) class has four isotypes
(IgG1, IgG2, IgG3, and IgG4) and the IgA class has two subclasses (IgA1 and IgA2). The IgD, IgM, and IgE classes are not usually subdivided.

58.Developing embryo is not rejected because of:
   a) Non expression of paternal antigen at 2 cell stage
   b) Absence of HLA A and B
   c) Presence of HLA G
   d) Immunity suppressor substance produce by endometrium
   e) All of above
      Answer: e

www.ingramcontent.com/pod-product-compliance
Lightning Source LLC
Chambersburg PA
CBHW080636180526
45168CB00008B/3196